# The Longevity Lifestyle

## Secrets to Living a Long and Healthy Life

William Copeland

# Table of Contents

# Introduction:

# Centenarians

A letter from Buckingham Palace is one of the great rewards for living to the age of 100 in England. This royal message goes out to every centenarian the palace hears about. Could that be a privilege you might live to experience? I should suggest that yes, it's very possible.

In fact, it's estimated that there were 15,120 centenarians in the UK alone in 2020, an increase of almost 18% from 2019 (Storey, 2021). The population division of the United Nations estimated that, worldwide, there were approximately 573,000 centenarians living in 2021 (Buchholz, 2021). Whether or not your goal is to make it to the 100 years club, everyone wants to live a long and healthy life. Even when you feel like you would rather do whatever you want without any consideration of possible consequences, you're doing so because you want a good life. We all have our own definition of what to consider a good life, but are those definitions always in line with what is truly best for us?

In life, it's always important to wonder if our habits are making us live more because they make us enjoy more experiences or live less because they shorten our lifespan. Sure, living until an advanced age is not necessarily a synonym for good health. For many people, living until a very old age while collecting a myriad of health issues along the way is not a very appealing objective. However, the goal is not simply to add more years to our biography but to keep ourselves in good shape during the process. The fact is people don't die of old age. They die from disease, and disease is, in almost every case, preventable or reversible.

Yes, I have said the unthinkable. It's not by chance, it's  not by fate, and it's not by  inheritance from your family. Almost all diseases are very preventable and reversible. Even in those cases when you feel like you acquired a disease by factors that are out of your control, with the right habits you can turn the tides, even if just by a little. In the world of healthcare, it's often said that prevention is more important than cure since there is no better way of saving someone from illness than by protecting them from the possibility of developing any disease in the first place.

Likewise, it's also often discussed how even the best surgeries and treatments need to be accompanied by the adoption of the right habits to fully guarantee successful results. Life does not necessarily have to be a race, but it can also be a marathon. With the right knowledge, you can turn your marathon into a walk that will make you live more in every sense of the word.

In this book, we will look at 3 simple areas of life that keep disease at bay and promote longevity so you can be confident that everything you're called to do will be fulfilled.

# Chapter 1

# Tiger in Our Midst—

# Understanding the Body's Stress

# Response

To understand our health and healing, we need to understand first something about the body that few people know and hardly any physician will teach.

Let me explain. Imagine I am driving a very sporty car that has two modes of operation. It has a regular driving mode and a sports mode. When my car is in regular mode, the engine and transmission are designed to respond very gently to the pressing of the gas pedal. When you press the pedal, the engine and transmission respond very slowly and quietly. However, in the sports mode, when I press the pedal, the engine goes *vroom* immediately. In this mode, the internals of the car are having very different responses to the pressure of the gas pedal.

Our bodies function just in the same way, also with two modes of operation. The two modes are called Fight or Flight and rest and digest. In order to dive deeper into this topic, we will need to look at an example from our ancestry.

Let's journey back many thousands of years to the days of the hunters and gatherers. Picture yourself out on a hunt for the day. As you sit down by the watering hole to take a drink, you notice two shimmering eyes peering at you from the brush. As your eyes adjust you recognize the silhouette of a tiger crouched to pounce. Your body at this point goes into a state called fight or flight—or, in scientific terms, the sympathetic nervous system response. This is a function of the Autonomic Nervous System and is an automatic response.

You may be thinking *what does this have to do with me staying healthy, fighting disease, and making it to the 100 years club?* Well, quite simply put, you can have your body in sports mode like my car some of the time but if you leave it on all the time your body will wear out quite quickly. It's very important we understand what states our bodies are in and how to control those states.

So let's look again at my old friend tiger crouching in the bushes. Nowadays, we typically don't have to expose ourselves to dangers such as tigers for daily endeavors, but we do have things that are just as scary. Every day, we're exposed to tigers like a traffic jam, work problems, and family difficulties. Our modern-day tigers are much more sophisticated problems than our ancient ancestors had, but our bodies can't tell the difference. When that unexpected bill comes in the mail, it might as well be a tiger jumping from the bush because your body perceives it in exactly the same manner. The fight or flight stage is activated!

Researchers have learned not only how this reaction occurs, but also what happens when you stay in a continual state of fight or flight. The body's stress response begins with our thoughts or the things we see. When you're confronted with a perceived danger your brain tells your adrenal glands to start sending out the hormone epinephrine, also known as adrenaline, into the bloodstream.

As adrenaline immediately circulates through the body, it causes a lot of changes to your body. One of the first changes happens in the heart, which starts to beat faster. In consequence, this gives extra blood to the muscles and vital organs. Blood pressure goes up and also breathing rate increases to give the body the extra alertness and energy needed to take immediate action. This whole process happens so fast that people usually do not realize the order in which said changes occur.

This is how people are able to respond to an emergency situation seemingly without even thinking. The sympathetic nervous system response is quite necessary for us, but here is where the real problem exists. If our brain stays in a state of perception-induced stress over a long period of time, the body begins a secondary continuation of the stress response. This continuation would be the adrenal glands releasing cortisol. As a result, your body then stays revved up on high alert.

While it's under the influence of said secondary continuation, the body will shut down digestion, diverting energy to places like muscles, and will also increase blood flow. People often have difficulty putting a stop to the stress response, which poses a problem. Continual states of even low-level stress can keep adrenal and cortisol levels high, putting your body in a continual state of overexertion—much like a car with the gas pedal pressed to the floor in sports mode. We could go on and on about the negative impacts of a constant state of stress but the real question is, how do we control our stress response and keep it from damaging our health?

In order to answer this question, we must take a closer look at building thought patterns. We may often feel like we cannot take some thoughts out of our heads but, as you'll see, the effects of these ruminations are anything but confined within our minds.

## The Physiology of Stress

Stress is an inevitable part of life. It can come from various sources such as work, family, relationships, or even the environment. While a small amount of stress can be helpful in motivating us to take action and perform better, chronic or severe stress can have a negative impact on our physical and mental health.

To understand the physiology of stress, we need to start with the nervous system. The nervous system is responsible for processing chemical and electrical signals that travel through our body at all times and allow us to do just about everything a human can do. From receiving information about the stimuli that surround us to responding to it, our nervous system is involved in everything, making the magic happen all the time!

The involvement of this complex and intricate network of structures and processes enables it to regulate and coordinate all of the body's functions. It plays a critical role in maintaining homeostasis, or balance, within the body, as well as in responding to changes in the external environment.

In order to participate in and regulate nearly all of our vital organs and processes, this complex system needs to function in a very organized way. Studies on the topic over the years have discovered that said organization begins with a fundamental division between the central and peripheral nervous system (Guy-Evans, 2021a).

Starting with the central nervous system, you can see it as the main center of control in the body. Being composed of the encephalon and the spinal cord, it serves as the main processing center for all incoming sensory information, as well as the center for the generation of motor responses. The brain is the most complex and magical organ in the human body. After all, it's literally the organ that studies itself since we simply would not be able to learn without it.

Our central nervous system is responsible for a wide range of functions, including consciousness, perception, memory, emotion, and movement. The spinal cord is a long, thin, tubular structure that runs from the brain down the length of the back. It serves as a pathway for communication between the brain and the rest of the body.

The peripheral nervous system is, as its name indicates, on the periphery of the central nervous system, reaching all the areas of the body that the central control unit cannot access directly. Composed of nerve fibers and ganglia, this system is further divided into two branches: the somatic nervous system and the autonomic nervous system. The former is responsible for controlling voluntary movements, while the latter is responsible for regulating involuntary functions such as heart rate, digestion, and respiration.

Within the central nervous system, there are several different divisions that play a role in regulating the body's response to stress. The limbic system, for example, is a group of structures located in the brain that is responsible for regulating emotions, including fear, anger, and anxiety. One of the key components of the limbic system is the amygdala, which is responsible for processing emotional stimuli and triggering the "fight or flight" response.

The hypothalamus is another key structure in the brain that is involved in the stress response. It's located near the base of the brain and plays a critical role in regulating a wide range of bodily functions, including hunger, thirst, body temperature, and sleep. It's also responsible for producing and releasing various hormones that play a role in the stress response, including cortisol and adrenaline.

Likewise, there are a group of structures known as the  basal ganglia that are located deep within the brain that are involved in a vast array of cognitive processes like, for example, the regulation of movement. They're also involved in the processing of emotions, particularly in response to rewarding stimuli. Dysfunction in the basal ganglia has been linked to a range of disorders, including Parkinson's disease and addiction.

Just like the nervous system as a whole can be partitioned into a central division and a peripheral division and each of these partitions has its own subsystem, each of these smaller divisions can be further divided into more functionally specific elements.

For example, the autonomic nervous system can also be divided into sympathetic and parasympathetic nervous systems as both of these divisions play a critical role in the overall work of the entire nervous system and the way it controls the body's response to stress. The sympathetic nervous system is responsible for triggering the "fight or flight" response, which prepares the body to respond to a perceived threat. This response is characterized by an increase in heart rate, respiration rate, and blood pressure, as well as the release of adrenaline and other stress hormones.

The parasympathetic nervous system, by contrast, is responsible for promoting relaxation and reducing the body's response to stress. It's responsible for slowing heart rate, reducing respiration rate, and promoting digestion and other functions associated with the "rest and digest" response.

When we encounter a stressor, such as a deadline at work or a difficult conversation, the nervous system kicks into action. The first part of the nervous system to respond is the sympathetic nervous system, which activates the "fight or flight" response.

The coordinated action of all the structures that conform our nervous system is what makes possible said *fight or flight* response by taking measures like, for example, preparing the body for action and releasing hormones such as adrenaline and noradrenaline, which increase heart rate, blood pressure, and respiration. These changes help us to be more alert and better able to respond to the source of stress.

As the stressor continues, the hypothalamus sends signals to a part of the brain that is as small as it is essential—the pituitary gland. Upon reception of said signals, this gland releases adrenocorticotropic hormone (ACTH). ACTH then travels to the adrenal glands, which are located on top of the kidneys. The adrenal glands release cortisol, a stress hormone, in response to the ACTH signal. Cortisol helps to regulate blood sugar levels and blood pressure, among other things, and also acts as an anti-inflammatory agent.

The release of cortisol is a crucial part of the stress response and is governed by the HPA axis. The HPA axis is a complex set of interactions between the hypothalamus, pituitary gland, and adrenal glands that regulate the body's response to stress. When the hypothalamus detects a stressor, it sends a signal to the pituitary gland to release ACTH, which, in turn, signals the adrenal glands to release cortisol.

The adrenal glands are one of the most important components of the body's stress response system. But why are they so important?

These small, triangular-shaped glands are located on top of each kidney and play a crucial role in regulating a wide range of bodily functions. These key glands aid the endocrine system in the production and release of hormones that regulate various physiological processes in the body. The adrenal glands are divided into two main parts: the adrenal cortex and the adrenal medulla. The adrenal cortex is responsible for the production of steroid hormones such as cortisol, aldosterone, and androgens, while the adrenal medulla is responsible for the production of catecholamines such as adrenaline and noradrenaline.

The adrenal glands play several important functions in the body, including the following:

- Helping the body respond to stress. One of the most important functions of the adrenal glands is to help the body respond to stress. When the body perceives a threat, the hypothalamus in the brain releases a hormone called corticotropin-releasing hormone (CRH), which triggers the pituitary gland to release adrenocorticotropic hormone (ACTH). ACTH, in turn, stimulates the adrenal glands to release cortisol and other stress hormones, which help the body respond to stress.

- Regulating blood pressure. The adrenal glands play a role in regulating blood pressure. The hormone aldosterone, which is produced in the adrenal cortex, helps regulate blood pressure by increasing the reabsorption of sodium and water in the kidneys, which leads to an increase in blood volume and blood pressure.

- Regulating blood sugar. The adrenal glands help to regulate blood sugar levels. The hormone cortisol, which is produced in the adrenal cortex, helps regulate blood sugar levels by increasing the breakdown of glycogen (stored glucose) in the liver and muscles and by decreasing glucose uptake by peripheral tissues.

- Regulating response to inflammation. The adrenal glands impact regulation of the body's response to inflammation. Cortisol, which is produced in the adrenal cortex, has anti-inflammatory properties and helps reduce inflammation in the body.

Being the interconnected family of systems and organs that it is, our body often works in a *butterfly-effect-esque* manner. In other words, changes in the levels of one substance usually affect others as well. This means that rises and drops in the level of cortisol also lead to variations in the levels of other important hormones that produce changes in our bodies, such as aldosterone, adrenaline, and noradrenaline.

Produced by the adrenal cortex, aldosterone helps regulate blood pressure by increasing the reabsorption of sodium and water in the kidneys, which leads to an increase in blood volume and blood pressure.

Adrenaline, also known as epinephrine, is a catecholamine produced by the adrenal medulla. It's released in response to stress and helps prepare the body for a fight-or-flight response by increasing heart rate, blood pressure, and respiration.

Noradrenaline, also known as norepinephrine, is a catecholamine produced by the adrenal medulla. It is released in response to stress and helps prepare the body for a fight-or-flight response by increasing heart rate, blood pressure, and respiration.

The HPA axis plays a vital role in our response to stress, but chronic stress can lead to dysregulation of the system, resulting in long-term health problems. When cortisol levels remain high for an extended period, it can lead to negative health effects, such as increased inflammation, decreased immune system function, and even changes to brain structure and function. These changes can increase the risk of chronic diseases such as depression, anxiety, heart disease, and diabetes.

It's essential to note that stress is not just a psychological phenomenon. It has a significant impact on the body, and its effects can be seen in various physiological processes. Chronic stress can lead to changes in the brain, including decreased neurogenesis, or the production of new neurons, in the hippocampus, a region of the brain involved in memory and emotion regulation. It can also lead to changes in the size of the amygdala, a region of the brain that plays a crucial role in our emotional responses.

In addition to the impact on the brain, chronic stress can also have significant effects on the immune system. Prolonged exposure to cortisol and other stress hormones can suppress the immune system, making us more vulnerable to infection and disease.

Stress can also affect the digestive system, leading to changes in appetite and digestion. It can cause an increase in stomach acid production, which can lead to gastrointestinal issues such as heartburn and acid reflux. Chronic stress has also been linked to the development of irritable bowel syndrome and inflammatory bowel disease.

## Chronic Stress and Its Effects on Health

Stress is a normal part of life, and in small doses it can even be beneficial. However, when stress becomes chronic, it can take a serious toll on both our physical and mental health. Chronic stress can result from ongoing challenges, such as work-related stress, relationship issues, or financial struggles.

As I said earlier, the effects of chronic stress on physical and mental health can reach far beyond the confines of our minds. In fact, our bodies are often just as affected as our minds. Chronic stress can have a vast array of effects on our bodies, but there are some that you'll need to pay more attention to than others.

One of the most fatal consequences that chronic stress can bring with it is an increased risk of heart disease and stroke. Stress activates the sympathetic nervous system in a way that can increase blood pressure, heart rate, and the risk of blood clots. Over time, these effects can take a toll on the cardiovascular system, increasing the risk of heart disease.

You may be wondering how exactly chronic stress can sicken our heart and make it more prone to suffer strokes. There are many ways in which the heart can get sick; knowing some of the most common ones may help you keep your stress from reaching very dangerous levels.

Cardiovascular disease is a broad term that encompasses several medical conditions that affect the heart and blood vessels. It's a leading cause of death worldwide, with an estimated 17.9 million deaths in 2019, according to the World Health Organization (*Cardiovascular diseases*, 2021). While there are several factors that can contribute to the development of cardiovascular disease, stress has been identified as a significant risk factor for several types of heart disease.

The most common types of cardiovascular disease include coronary artery disease, heart failure, stroke, and arrhythmia.

- Coronary artery disease (CAD) is the most common type of heart disease and occurs when the arteries that supply blood to the heart become narrowed or blocked. Besides the risk of stroke, this type of disease is commonly seen causing people chest pains and even shortness of breath.

- Heart failure occurs when the heart is unable to pump enough blood to meet the body's needs, which can lead to fatigue, shortness of breath, and swelling in the legs and feet.

- Stroke occurs when a blood vessel that supplies the brain is blocked or ruptures, which can lead to the loss of brain function, disability, or death.

- Arrhythmia refers to an irregular heartbeat that can cause the heart to beat too fast, too slow, or in an irregular pattern.

Cardiovascular disease can be caused by a variety of factors, including genetics, lifestyle, and environmental factors. While some factors, such as genetics, are beyond our control, there are steps we can take to reduce the risk of heart disease, such as maintaining a healthy weight, exercising regularly, and managing stress.

Stress can also cause illnesses related to hormonal imbalances such as increased heart rate, blood pressure, and blood sugar levels. Over time, these changes can damage the arteries and lead to the development of plaque, which can narrow the arteries and increase the risk of a heart attack. In addition, stress can lead to unhealthy behaviors, such as overeating and a lack of physical activity, which can contribute to the development of heart failure.

Chronic stress can also affect the immune system, making it more difficult for the body to fight off infections and diseases. Stress hormones such as cortisol can suppress the immune system, leaving the body more vulnerable to illnesses.

The immune system is a complex network of cells, tissues, and organs that work together to protect the body from harmful pathogens such as bacteria, viruses, and fungi. The immune system is a crucial component of our overall health and well-being, and it helps to prevent us from becoming ill.

The immune system can be divided into two main components: the innate immune system and the adaptive immune system.

The innate immune system is the first line of defense against foreign invaders. It consists of physical barriers such as the skin and mucous membranes, as well as cells such as neutrophils and macrophages. These cells are able to identify and eliminate pathogens without prior exposure to them.

The adaptive immune system is more complex than the innate immune system and takes longer to develop a response. This system consists of white blood cells known as lymphocytes, including B cells and T cells, which are able to recognize and remember specific pathogens. When the body is exposed to a new pathogen, the adaptive immune system mounts a response to eliminate the invader and prevent future infections. This response is known as the immune response, and it involves the production of antibodies and the activation of immune cells.

As you can see, the immune response is beyond critical for protecting the body against a wide range of infections and diseases. Stress can have a negative impact on the immune system, and it can cause a range of immune deficiency symptoms. Some of the most common immune deficiency symptoms caused by stress include:

- Lower white blood cell count. One of the most significant effects of stress on the immune system is a decrease in the number of white blood cells. White blood cells are a crucial component of the immune system, and they're responsible for fighting off infections and diseases. When the number of white blood cells decreases, the body is more susceptible to infections and illnesses.

- Chronic inflammation. Inflammation is a normal response to injury or infection, and it's an important part of the immune system's response. However, chronic inflammation can lead to tissue damage and increase the risk of a range of diseases, including heart disease, diabetes, and cancer. Stress can increase the level of inflammation in the body, which can contribute to the development of these diseases.

- Infections. When the immune system is compromised, the body is more susceptible to infections. Stress can weaken the immune system, making it easier for pathogens to invade the body and cause illness.

- Autoimmune disease. In the case of autoimmune diseases, stress can increase the risk of them happening by causing the immune system to see the healthy cells as targets and attack them.

Remember that while immune system deficiency has not been proven to directly cause many of the aforementioned diseases, it can certainly leave your body more likely to develop and be severely affected by them.

Chronic stress is a major risk factor for the development of mental health disorders such as anxiety and depression. This is because stress can alter the balance of chemicals in the brain, making it more difficult to regulate emotions and causing feelings of sadness, anxiety, and irritability.

Chronic stress can also lead to a host of digestive issues such as irritable bowel syndrome, stomach ulcers, and acid reflux. Stress can affect the way the digestive system works, causing symptoms such as nausea, stomach pain, and diarrhea.

It's important to note that these are just a few of the many ways that chronic stress can impact our health. When stress becomes chronic, it can affect nearly every system in the body, increasing the risk of a wide range of physical and mental health issues.

# Recognizing Signs of Stress Overload

When stress becomes chronic, it can take a significant toll on our physical and mental health. This is known as stress overload, and it is something that is becoming increasingly common in today's world.

Said stress overload occurs when the demands of our environment overwhelm us to the point of making us feel like we can no longer cope with our daily challenges. This can happen in any area of our lives, from work and relationships to financial pressures and health concerns. Stress overload can disrupt our capabilities to function efficiently every day with such ease because it can appear in a number of different ways, including sleep disturbance, muscle tension, and irritability.

Identifying stress overload can become quite a hard task when we're already going through it and our mind feels full of noisy and chaotic thoughts. However, the process can become at least a little bit easier if we know what signs to look for.

One of the main habits you should adopt as soon as possible is paying attention to your sleep patterns. If you're having trouble falling or staying asleep, it could be a sign that your stress levels are too high. Stress can interfere with the natural sleep cycle, making it difficult to get the rest you need to function at your best.

Similarly, you may also want to get familiar with and monitor your muscle tension. When we're under stress, our muscles tend to tighten up as part of the fight-or-flight response. If you notice that you're constantly clenching your jaw, tensing your shoulders, or experiencing headaches, it could be a sign that you're experiencing stress overload.

Achieving and maintaining a good connection with your emotions is key to any form of self-care you want to apply in life. Stress can make us more irritable or emotional than usual. If you find yourself snapping at others, feeling on edge, or experiencing mood swings, it may be a sign that you're experiencing stress overload.

To record the results of your efforts, you may also want to take note of physical symptoms. Chronic stress can manifest in a variety of physical symptoms, including digestive issues, headaches, and even heart palpitations. If you notice any of these symptoms, it's important to take them seriously and seek support.

## Lessons Learned Along the Way

When we think of stress, we usually think of it as a mental process or as a feeling not so different from the likes of sadness or frustration. However, the truth is that almost all of our emotions happen at both a physiological and a mental level.

The aforementioned mind and body dualism can go from the natural and necessary process of having our neurons fire neurotransmitters when we think to the dangerous process of having our physical health decline as much—or even more—than our mental well-being as a product of high doses of stress.

It's often the case that, to study just how powerful and devastating the effects of chronic stress can be, we just have to look at our own lives. That is what I did, and it certainly taught me a lesson.

Nowadays, I can see up close and personally that going wholeheartedly after your dreams gives life to your soul, while giving up on your dreams and quitting your calling dries you to the bone. However, that has not always been the case. In fact, I never fully understood the weight of these words until my journey as a business owner started to take a toll on my health.

Growing up, I always knew that I wanted to own my own commercial printing business. Seeing millions of printed pieces rolling off the press cut, folded, packaged, and shipped to customers all over the country made me believe that anything was possible. And in November of 2009, my dream finally became a reality. My very own printing press was being unloaded ever so carefully, and the excitement was palpable. But what I didn't know was that the endless nights of work and the non-stop pressure would soon take a toll on my health.

As a young man in my late twenties, I thought I was invincible. I could work for 80 hours a week, get only four to five hours of sleep at night, and survive on endless cups of coffee. I believed that I didn't need to worry about stress management, diet, or physical exercise. All I needed was to work and run all day long.

But as the years went by, I started to notice the toll that this lifestyle was taking on me. I became a constant whirlwind, always on the go and at work all the time. And before I knew it, I started to break down mentally and physically.

In 2016, I hit my bottom. I was experiencing a high level of anxiety, which turned into panic attacks and various random health problems. I realized that something was not working, but I had no idea what was wrong. I didn't know that stress levels affect your emotional and physical health. I didn't know that diet and exercise play such a vital role in our longevity. I thought that if you had any problems, you just went to the doctor and took a pill for whatever was wrong.

But the truth is, we can take control of our own health. We don't have to mindlessly take any medication that is thrown at us. We can manage our stress levels, discipline our diets, and take joy in strengthening our bodies through movement and physical training. The Bible tells us that we're fearfully and wonderfully made, and our minds and bodies have great power to heal, recover, and be in a state of great power.

## Managing Stress Mindfulness and Self-Care

It's important to take care of ourselves and manage stress so that we can live a healthy and fulfilling life. This essentially means adopting the habit of self-care which is the practice of taking care of yourself physically, mentally, and emotionally.

Finding ways to prioritize your well-being and manage stress in a healthy and sustainable way can turn your life around for the better, but you need to know how to do it. There are many different strategies for self-care, and what works for one person might not work for another. But the important thing is to find what works for you and to make it a regular part of your routine.

One effective strategy for managing stress through self-care is mindfulness. Mindfulness is the practice of being present in the moment and aware of your thoughts and feelings without judgment. It's about being in the moment and focusing on what's happening right now, rather than worrying about the past or future.

Another effective strategy for self-care is exercise. Exercise is a powerful way to manage stress because it helps to release endorphins, which are natural mood-boosters. Even just 20-30 minutes of exercise per day can help to reduce stress and improve your overall sense of well-being.

Deep breathing is another simple but effective strategy for managing stress through self-care. Deep breathing exercises can help to calm your mind and body, reduce muscle tension, and promote relaxation. To practice deep breathing, simply take a deep breath in through your nose, hold it for a few seconds, and then exhale slowly through your mouth. Repeat this for several minutes until you feel more relaxed and calm.

While you're practicing deep breathing, you can boost its effects by slowly tensing and then relaxing different muscle groups in your body. Just make sure that you follow an order that allows you to work on just a few muscles at a time. This technique, known as progressive muscle relaxation, can help you become more aware of your body and release tension that you might not even realize you're holding. To practice progressive muscle relaxation, start by tensing the muscles in your toes, then your feet, your legs, and so on, until you've tensed and relaxed every muscle group in your body.

In addition to these strategies, there are many other ways to practice self-care and manage stress. For example, you might try taking a relaxing bath, getting a massage, or spending time in nature. You might also find it helpful to journal, practice yoga or meditation, or spend time with loved ones.

The key to self-care is to make it a regular part of your routine. It's not something that you can do once in a while and expect to see results. Instead, it's something that you need to prioritize and make time for every day. Even just a few minutes of self-care each day can make a big difference in how you feel and how you manage stress.

# Chapter 2:

# Cycles—Understanding the Connection Between Thoughts and Stress

I know you have heard the phrase "mind over matter" and, despite seeming a little too ideological, it's actually true. Our thoughts create matter!

When we produce a thought, the outcome of that action actually holds space in our brain. Neural pathways and proteins are produced when we think. Scientists have studied these pathways in our brains and have compared them to real-life paths like the ones we would see in a forest.

Have you ever been on a walking trail in the woods? If so, have you noticed that when many people travel the same path constantly, it becomes worn down and easy to follow? Conversely, what if a path has been less traveled? The trail can often be overgrown and hard to pass through.

That is exactly how our brain works. As we come up with different thoughts, they produce pathways. As we consistently produce the same thoughts, their corresponding pathways become more defined and more easily traveled.

This means that if a certain thought comes to your mind frequently, its pathway will become well-traveled, making it easier and easier for you to think about it again. In other words, this whole process is like a habit or a continuous cycle that can become quite hard to break out of. After all, it disrupts the one tool that we will need to break free: *our way of thinking.*

That is why if we rehearse over and over again a stressful thought pattern, we will start to gravitate to this way of thinking subconsciously and automatically. Our brains can get stuck in a non-stop loop of stressful thoughts. As these paths made of worries are traveled over and over again, our body keeps listening as it's being told to move into the fight or flight state.

Just as we can make neural pathways of fear, anxiety, and stress in our brains, we can also carve out thought pathways of joy, delight, and peace. Developing these healthy thought patterns can help us develop a style of thinking that we will be subconsciously drawn to, moving our minds automatically toward positive states of well-being.

Training your mind on what path to follow can mean all the difference in the world regarding the state in which our body will remain. You can either learn to navigate toward a state of fight or flight or learn to steer clear of it and find the state of rest and digest.

As we explore longevity and health in this book, we must understand that maintaining a healthy thought pattern in our minds is essential to keeping our bodies in good shape. When we keep the right mindset, we give our bodies the state of rest that they need to heal and increase their chances of successfully fighting off diseases.

## The Chemical Response to Thoughts

As we go through our day-to-day lives, our thoughts can significantly impact our emotional and physical well-being. The chemical processes of our brains determine how we react to stressors, both positive and negative, and this has a powerful impact on our health.

Let's begin by remembering the hormones involved in the body's stress response. Keep in mind that the hypothalamus-pituitary-adrenal (HPA) axis is a major system in the body that regulates stress. One of the main functions of this circuit is to regulate the processing of cortisol in our body. Cortisol is an essential hormone that can be very essential in helping the body cope with stress; however, chronically high cortisol levels can lead to negative health outcomes such as anxiety, depression, and metabolic disorders.

When we think of stress, we often think of how it affects us emotionally and physically, but we don't always consider how it affects our neurological processes. However, stress can significantly impact the way we think, both in the short and long term.

It's essential to understand that thinking is a complex process that involves several brain structures and systems. At the core of this process is the limbic system, which is a group of brain structures that includes the amygdala, hippocampus, and hypothalamus. These structures work together to regulate emotions, memories, and physiological responses.

The amygdala, for instance, is responsible for processing emotions, particularly fear and anxiety. It helps us to identify potential threats in our environment and activate the appropriate physiological responses to deal with them. The hippocampus plays a critical role in the formation and retrieval of memories, while the hypothalamus regulates several physiological functions, such as appetite, thirst, and body temperature.

Another essential brain structure involved in thinking is the prefrontal cortex. This part of the brain is responsible for executive functions, such as planning, decision-making, and impulse control. It's also involved in regulating emotions and social behavior.

The prefrontal cortex works in conjunction with the limbic system to process information and generate responses. When the brain is functioning optimally, the prefrontal cortex balances the emotional responses generated by the limbic system, allowing us to make rational decisions based on the situation at hand. However, stress can disrupt this balance, leading to cognitive impairments and emotional dysregulation.

One way that stress can impact our cognitive abilities is by altering the structural and functional connectivity of the brain. Chronic stress, in particular, has been linked to the shrinkage of brain regions associated with cognitive executive functions, such as the prefrontal cortex and the hippocampus. This shrinkage can lead to impairments in memory, attention, and decision-making.

Additionally, stress can affect the communication between the limbic system and the prefrontal cortex, leading to emotional dysregulation. For instance, under conditions of high stress, the amygdala can override the prefrontal cortex, leading to impulsive behaviors and emotional outbursts.

When you zoom past the point of structures, you discover that, in the brain, the magic happens thanks to neurotransmitters. These tiny substances can be seen as the protagonists of the communication between our brain structures.

Given their many functions, simply saying that neurotransmitters are involved in our thoughts and stress response would be an understatement. Dopamine, norepinephrine, serotonin, and GABA are four essential neurotransmitters that play a crucial role in regulating our emotions, thoughts, and physical response to stress. Dopamine and norepinephrine are involved in our body's "fight or flight" response and can lead to feelings of anxiety and stress when released in high amounts. Serotonin is known for its role in regulating mood, and low levels of serotonin can lead to depression and anxiety. GABA, on the other hand, is an inhibitory neurotransmitter that can help reduce anxiety and promote feelings of calmness and relaxation.

Now that we understand the hormones and neurotransmitters involved in our stress response, let's explore how our thoughts can lead to relaxation or stress. Positive thoughts and emotions can help stimulate the release of dopamine, serotonin, and GABA, leading to feelings of relaxation and happiness. On the other hand, negative thoughts and emotions can trigger the release of cortisol and norepinephrine, leading to feelings of stress and anxiety.

The brain is a powerful tool that can help us manage stress and promote relaxation. By learning to control our thoughts, we can effectively manage stress and reduce the negative impact it can have on our health. Mindfulness and meditation can be effective tools for controlling our thoughts and emotions, promoting relaxation and reducing stress.

# The Power of Thoughts in Regulating Stress

While this stress response is necessary for survival, chronic stress can cause problems. One of the main consequences of chronic stress is an increase in cortisol levels. When cortisol levels remain high for extended periods of time, it can lead to a decrease in immune function, making us more susceptible to illness and disease. Additionally, high levels of cortisol can cause a host of other physical problems, such as weight gain, high blood pressure, and impaired glucose metabolism.

But the severity of our stress response isn't just determined by the presence of a stressor or the amount of stress we're experiencing. It's also influenced by our thoughts and attitudes towards the stressor. For example, if we view a work deadline as a challenge that we're capable of meeting, we're likely to experience less stress than if we view it as an insurmountable obstacle. Our thoughts and attitudes can influence our perception of stress, and ultimately, our physical response to it.

In addition to our thoughts and attitudes, our social environment can also impact the severity of our stress response. Research has shown that individuals who experience chronic stress in the context of a supportive social network tend to have lower levels of cortisol than those who experience chronic stress in the absence of social support. This underscores the importance of social connections in managing stress and maintaining good health.

Our diet can also play a role in the severity of our stress response. Consuming a diet high in processed foods and refined sugars can increase inflammation in the body, making us more vulnerable to the negative effects of chronic stress. By contrast, a diet rich in fruits, vegetables, whole grains, and lean protein can help to reduce inflammation and support healthy immune function.

# Incorporating Positive Thoughts into Daily Life

Negative thoughts can be toxic and cause stress to build up in our bodies. We all experience negative thoughts at some point, but it's important to recognize when they're becoming a pattern and affecting our mental and physical health. The first step to reducing negative thoughts is to become aware of them. Take some time to reflect on the thoughts that go through your mind and try to identify any recurring negative patterns.

Meditation is a powerful tool to reduce negative thoughts and promote positive thinking. By practicing mindfulness meditation, we can learn to observe our thoughts without judgment and let them pass by without getting caught up in them. This can help to break the cycle of negative thinking and promote a more positive outlook on life. Guided meditations can be found online or through meditation apps and can help beginners learn the basics of mindfulness meditation.

Cognitive reframing is another technique to reduce negative thoughts and promote positive thinking. It involves recognizing and challenging negative thoughts and replacing them with more positive ones. For example, if you find yourself thinking *I'll never be able to do this*, try reframing it as *This is challenging, but I can learn and improve with practice.* This technique takes practice but can be extremely effective in shifting your perspective and reducing stress.

Our life narratives can also impact our thoughts and attitudes. These can be seen as mental representations that we have about ourselves and that come in the form of stories. We all have a sort of self-biography in our minds that contains our strengths, weaknesses, and essentially the way in which we perceive ourselves.

If your life narrative is primarily negative, it can be difficult to break the cycle of negative thinking. Take some time to reflect on your life narrative and try to identify any negative patterns. Then, work to rewrite your life narrative in a more positive light. Focus on your strengths, accomplishments, and positive experiences.

Incorporating positive thoughts into our daily lives takes practice and effort, but it can have a profound impact on our mental and physical health. By reducing negative thoughts, we can reduce stress and improve our overall well-being. So, take some time each day to reflect on your thoughts, practice mindfulness meditation, challenge negative thoughts with cognitive reframing, and rewrite your life narrative in a more positive light.

# Takeaways

We've explored the brain chemical processes underlying our thoughts and how they impact our stress response, and we learned how negative thinking can have a severe effect on our overall well-being.

But there is good news! We have the power to shift our thinking and develop consistently positive thought patterns that lead to relaxation, resilience, and better health outcomes. By incorporating meditation, cognitive reframing, and creating new life narratives, we can reduce the negative thoughts that contribute to stress and anxiety.

It's important to remember that developing positive thought patterns takes time and effort, just like building any other skill or habit. But the benefits are significant and long-lasting. We can improve our immune function, decrease our risk of chronic diseases, and increase our overall sense of happiness and wellbeing.

It's worth noting that positive thinking doesn't mean ignoring the challenges and difficulties we face in life. Instead, it means approaching these challenges with a mindset of growth and resilience, finding opportunities for learning and growth even in the face of adversity.

As we move forward in our journey to manage stress and improve our overall health, let's keep in mind the power of our thoughts and attitudes. Let's commit to developing positive thought patterns and consistently nurturing our mental and emotional wellbeing. And let's remember that, with practice, we can all cultivate a more positive and fulfilling life.

Chapter 3:

# New Paths in the Forest—

# Understanding the Power of

# Thoughts and Habits

We all know that our thoughts have a significant impact on our overall well-being. Negative thoughts and patterns can lead to stress, anxiety, and even physical health problems. By contrast, positive thoughts and patterns can help us feel more calm, confident, and content.

Meditation is a powerful tool for cultivating positive thought patterns. When we meditate, we slow down our minds and become more aware of our thoughts. This heightened awareness allows us to observe our thoughts without getting caught up in them. Over time, we can begin to replace negative thought patterns with positive ones.

Research has shown that people who have a positive outlook on life are more likely to enjoy better physical health, recover from illness more quickly, and even live longer. Positive thinking can also reduce stress levels and improve our overall quality of life.

But how do we create positive thought patterns through meditation? The key is to focus on positive thoughts and emotions during our meditation practice. We can do this by visualizing positive outcomes, repeating affirmations, or simply focusing on feelings of gratitude, joy, or love.

It's important to remember that creating positive thought patterns takes time and consistent effort. Just like going to the gym, we need to make meditation a regular part of our routine if we want to see results. But with patience and practice, we can rewire our brains and create new, more positive thought patterns that serve us well.

## The Connection Between Thoughts and Habits

Have you ever noticed that you tend to repeat the same patterns of behavior over and over again? Maybe you have a habit of procrastinating, or you always turn to junk food when you're feeling stressed. Whatever the case may be, our habits are closely linked to our thoughts.

In fact, our thoughts can have a profound impact on the development of habits. The brain is constantly forming neural pathways based on our experiences and behaviors. The more frequently we repeat a behavior, the stronger the neural pathway becomes. And our thoughts play a key role in shaping these pathways.

When we have a thought, it triggers a chain reaction in the brain. The brain releases neurotransmitters, which are chemical messengers that send signals to other parts of the brain and body. These neurotransmitters help to create and strengthen the neural pathways that underlie our habits.

For example, let's say you have a thought that you're not good enough. This thought triggers the release of cortisol, a stress hormone that is associated with negative emotions. Over time, the repetition of this thought can create a neural pathway that is linked to feelings of low self-esteem and self-doubt.

Similarly, positive thoughts can also shape our habits. When we have a positive thought, the brain releases dopamine, a neurotransmitter that is associated with pleasure and reward. The more frequently we have positive thoughts, the stronger the neural pathways become that are linked to positive emotions and behaviors.

So, if you want to develop healthy habits, it's important to focus on cultivating positive thoughts. This doesn't mean that you should ignore negative thoughts or emotions. Rather, it means that you should be mindful of your thoughts and actively work to reframe negative thoughts into positive ones.

Thanks to a certain  ability every human brain is born with, we're able to use positive thoughts to our advantage and shape the way in which we consistently perceive things. The endless possibilities for getting our minds used to a certain style of thinking come from a phenomenon called neuroplasticity.

Neuroplasticity, also known as brain plasticity, is the brain's ability to change and reorganize itself in response to various experiences. It's a fascinating and ever-evolving area of neuroscience that has important implications for our ability to learn, adapt, and recover from injury or trauma.

At its core, brain plasticity refers to the brain's ability to form new connections between neurons and modify existing ones in response to changes in the environment or experiences. This occurs through the process of neural plasticity, which involves changes in the strength and connectivity of synapses, the spaces between neurons that allow them to communicate with one another.

The process of brain plasticity is driven by a variety of factors, including genetic and epigenetic influences, experiences and environmental factors, and various cellular and molecular mechanisms. One key mechanism that underlies plasticity is the activation of neural growth factors, which are proteins that promote the growth, survival, and differentiation of neurons.

There are several different types of neural growth factors, each with its own unique functions and effects on the brain.

## *Brain-Derived Neurotrophic Factor (BDNF)*

BDNF is perhaps the most well-known and extensively studied neural growth factor. It plays a crucial role in promoting the growth and survival of neurons, particularly in the hippocampus and cortex, which are regions of the brain involved in learning and memory.

Research has shown that BDNF is involved in various aspects of brain plasticity, including the formation and maintenance of new synapses, the growth of dendrites (the branched extensions of neurons that receive signals from other cells), and the regulation of gene expression in response to experiences.

BDNF is also thought to play a role in mediating the effects of stress on the brain. Stressful experiences can reduce BDNF levels, which may contribute to the development of depression, anxiety, and other mood disorders. Conversely, exercise, cognitive stimulation, and other forms of positive experiences can increase BDNF levels and promote brain plasticity.

## *Nerve Growth Factor (NGF)*

NGF is another important neural growth factor that plays a key role in the development and maintenance of the nervous system. It's involved in promoting the growth and survival of sensory neurons, as well as the development and function of the sympathetic and parasympathetic nervous systems.

In addition to its developmental roles, NGF impacts adult brain plasticity, particularly in the areas of learning and memory. Studies have shown that NGF can enhance the survival of newly generated neurons in the hippocampus, which is important for maintaining cognitive function throughout life.

## *Insulin-Like Growth Factor (IGF-1)*

IGF-1 is a hormone that plays a crucial role in regulating growth and development throughout the body. In the brain, IGF-1 is involved in promoting the growth and survival of neurons, as well as the formation and maintenance of synapses.

Research has shown that IGF-1 is particularly important for promoting brain plasticity in response to exercise and other forms of physical activity. Exercise has been shown to increase IGF-1 levels in the brain, which in turn promotes the growth of new neurons and synapses, as well as the survival of existing ones.

### *N-Methyl-D-Aspartate Receptors (NMDARs)*

NMDARs are a type of receptor found on the surface of neurons that are involved in the regulation of synaptic plasticity. They play a key role in mediating the effects of glutamate, a neurotransmitter that is involved in a variety of important functions, including learning and memory.

Insulin processing, sensory processing, and even neural growth induced by the experiences that our brain is exposed to on repeated occasions. As you may have guessed by now, stress has the power to interfere with each and every single one of these processes. So, one of the wisest decisions you can make is to embrace the impact that positive thoughts can have on your health.

# The Impact of Positive Thoughts on Health

Have you ever heard the phrase "think positive"? You might be surprised to know that there's more to this saying than just a feel-good message. In fact, positive thoughts can have a significant impact on your health—both physical and mental.

Our thoughts and attitudes play a crucial role in determining our well-being. Positive thoughts can lead to reduced stress, better mood, and improved physical health. Negative thoughts, on the other hand, can lead to increased stress, anxiety, and even physical health problems.

One of the most significant benefits of positive thinking is reduced stress. When we have positive thoughts, our bodies release hormones like dopamine and serotonin that create a sense of well-being and happiness. These hormones can help reduce stress levels and make us more resilient in the face of stressors.

Furthermore, positive thinking can help us maintain a healthy immune system. Studies have shown that negative emotions can suppress the immune system, making us more susceptible to illnesses. Conversely, positive emotions can boost the immune system, making us more resistant to illnesses.

In addition to its physical benefits, positive thinking has benefits for mental well-being. When we have a positive outlook on life, we're more likely to have better self-esteem, be more motivated, and have a greater sense of purpose. Positive thoughts can help us overcome negative experiences and even improve symptoms of mental health disorders like depression and anxiety.

Another positive way in which our thoughts can influence our behavior is by motivating us to adopt healthy habits like exercising more and eating better. These habits can, in turn, reduce the risk of chronic diseases like heart disease, diabetes, and obesity.

It's important to note that positive thinking is not about ignoring or denying negative emotions. Rather, it's about acknowledging negative thoughts and emotions while choosing to focus on the positive aspects of a situation. It's about developing a mindset that allows us to see opportunities instead of obstacles and solutions instead of problems.

## The Impact of Negative Thoughts on Health

Negative thoughts can have a significant impact on our health and well-being, and we often underestimate the power they hold over us. The reality is that our thoughts can affect our physical health as well as our mental state. The way we think and the things we tell ourselves can influence our emotions, behavior, and even our health.

When we experience negative thoughts, our bodies release stress hormones such as cortisol, adrenaline, and noradrenaline, which trigger the fight-or-flight response. While this response can be useful in some situations, such as when we need to react quickly to a dangerous situation, it can be harmful when experienced chronically. Chronic stress can lead to a weakened immune system, cardiovascular problems, and other health issues.

Negative thoughts can also contribute to mental health disorders such as anxiety and depression. When we focus on negative thoughts, we can easily fall into a pattern of rumination, where we repeatedly dwell on negative events, causing feelings of helplessness and hopelessness.

The effects of negative thinking can also impact our behavior. When we feel down or anxious, we may be less likely to engage in activities that could make us feel better, such as exercising or socializing with friends. We may also turn to unhealthy coping mechanisms, such as overeating or drinking alcohol, which can further exacerbate our negative feelings.

The link between negative thinking and physical and mental health is not always immediately apparent, but it's a well-documented phenomenon. Research has shown that people who have a more negative outlook on life are at a higher risk of developing a range of health problems, from heart disease to depression.

# Developing Positive Thought Patterns and Habits

As we've discussed earlier, our thoughts play a crucial role in shaping our behaviors and emotions, and they can also have a profound impact on our physical and mental health. Negative thoughts can increase stress, depression, and anxiety, while positive thoughts can enhance our mood, reduce stress, and improve immune function.

Fortunately, you can learn to develop positive thought patterns and habits, which can help you to promote your health and well-being. To do that, you'll need to become your best ally. When you take a look inside your mind, you may find the turmoil of disorganized negative thoughts. However, diving deep inside your mind and your heart can also provide you with all the optimism you may need.

One of the best ways to cultivate positive thinking is through journaling. By writing down our thoughts and feelings, we can gain clarity about our emotions and work through any negative thought patterns that may be affecting us. You can write about anything that comes to your mind, such as your day's events, your goals, your emotions, or your achievements. Try to focus on the good things that happened in your day, no matter how small they may seem. This practice can help you to shift your focus from negative to positive thoughts and make you feel more positive.

Visualization is another powerful tool that can help you to cultivate positive thoughts and develop positive habits. This practice involves picturing yourself achieving your goals or having a positive experience, in as much detail as possible. By visualizing your success or happiness, you can program your subconscious mind to work towards achieving your goals or experiencing positive outcomes.

Similarly, practicing gratitude can help you to focus on the positive aspects of your life and shift your focus away from negative thoughts. You can do this by taking a few minutes each day to reflect on the things you're grateful for, such as your health, your family, your friends, or even the small things like a beautiful sunset or a delicious meal. By focusing on the positive things in your life, you can cultivate a more positive outlook and reduce stress and anxiety.

Positive affirmations can also help you stay healthy as they're positive statements that you repeat to yourself regularly. These statements can be about yourself, your life, or your goals, and they can help to reinforce positive thinking patterns. You can say things like *I am capable of achieving my goals* or *I am worthy of love and happiness*. By repeating positive affirmations to yourself regularly, you can reprogram your mind to focus on the positive aspects of your life.

Even when you feel you're not doing very well at taking care of yourself, remember the importance of compassion. Self-compassion is one of the most valuable habits you can adopt. This means being kind and understanding towards yourself, just as you would be towards a friend or loved one. You can practice self-compassion by speaking to yourself kindly, forgiving yourself for mistakes, and treating yourself with the same love and respect that you give to others. By practicing self-compassion, you can develop a more positive outlook and reduce negative self-talk.

## Takeaways

It's  no secret to anyone that our thoughts and attitudes are incredibly powerful and can influence our behaviors, habits, and ultimately, our health. Developing positive thought patterns and habits can help reduce stress, increase feelings of happiness and well-being, and even boost our immune system.

We've also seen how negative thinking can have the opposite effect, leading to increased stress, depression, and anxiety. But the good news is that we can change our thought patterns and create new neural pathways in the brain, allowing us to break free from negative thinking and create more positive habits and behaviors.

By incorporating simple, practical strategies such as journaling, visualization of good scenarios, and gratitude practices, we can begin to reframe our thoughts and shift our focus to the positive aspects of our lives.

Remember, developing positive thought patterns and habits is a journey, not a destination. It takes time and effort, but the benefits to our health and well-being are well worth it. So, let's commit to nurturing positive thoughts and habits in our daily lives and enjoy the many benefits that come with it.

# Chapter 4:

# The American Diet Disaster—How Busy Lifestyles and Poor Food Choices are Fueling Chronic Diseases

The standard American diet, also known as SAD, is a diet that is high in processed foods, refined sugars, and unhealthy fats. It's a diet that's low in whole, nutrient-dense foods like fruits, vegetables, and whole grains. This type of diet is the norm for many Americans and has become a major contributor to a variety of health problems.

One of the most significant impacts of the standard American diet is its role in the rise of chronic diseases like obesity, diabetes, and heart disease. The high levels of processed and refined foods in this diet can lead to a variety of health problems, including inflammation, insulin resistance, and high cholesterol. Over time, these conditions can develop into chronic diseases that significantly impact our quality of life.

Our diet is not only impacting our physical health but also our mental health. Studies have shown that consuming a diet high in sugar and processed foods can lead to depression, anxiety, and other mental health issues. In contrast, a diet high in whole, nutrient-dense foods like fruits and vegetables can lead to better mental health outcomes.

While the standard American diet may seem like the easiest and most convenient option, it's clear that it's not serving us well. It's time for us to take a closer look at what we're putting into our bodies and make a change for the better.

## The American Diet: What Is Wrong With It?

Many of us are familiar with the term "American diet," and it's not something to brag about. The American diet refers to a style of eating that's characterized by high consumption of processed foods, unhealthy fats, added sugars, and animal products, as well as low intake of essential nutrients and fiber. This style of eating is not only unhealthy but also dangerous, as it can lead to many imbalances in the body that result in inflammation and disease.

One of the primary problems with the American diet is that it's filled with highly processed foods. These foods are usually high in sugar, unhealthy fats, and salt, and low in essential nutrients, including fiber, vitamins, and minerals. In other words, they're not really "food" in the sense that our bodies need them to function optimally. Eating a diet high in processed foods can lead to weight gain, diabetes, heart disease, and other chronic health conditions.

Another major problem with the American diet is the overconsumption of unhealthy fats. Trans fats and saturated fats are abundant in the American diet, and these fats can lead to inflammation, heart disease, and other health problems. They're found in many processed foods, fast foods, and fried foods, which are all staples of the American diet.

Added sugars are another significant problem with the American diet. Sugary drinks, candy, and desserts are everywhere, and they're a major source of empty calories. They contribute to weight gain, insulin resistance, and other health issues. The average American consumes more than 17 teaspoons of added sugar per day, which is far above the recommended limit of six teaspoons per day for women and nine teaspoons per day for men.

Finally, the American diet is high in animal products, including meat, dairy, and eggs. While these foods can provide essential nutrients, they're also high in saturated fat and can contribute to chronic health problems. In addition, the production of animal products is a major source of greenhouse gas emissions and contributes to environmental degradation.

When we eat a diet that's high in processed foods, unhealthy fats, added sugars, and animal products, we're not giving our bodies the nutrients they need to function properly. As a result, we may experience inflammation, which can lead to many chronic health conditions, including heart disease, diabetes, and cancer. To avoid the negative consequences of the American diet, it's important to focus on consuming a variety of whole, plant-based foods.

The meaning of plant based is, in fact, quite simple. It refers to foods such as fruits, vegetables, whole grains, legumes, nuts, seeds, and the like that originate straight from plants with as little processing as possible before they end up on your plate. These types of foods are high in fiber, vitamins, minerals, and antioxidants, which can protect against inflammation and disease.

When we consume whole, plant-based foods, we can also reduce our intake of unhealthy fats and added sugars. Further, we can reduce our environmental impact by reducing our consumption of animal products. By making these dietary changes, we can improve our health, protect the environment, and feel better overall.

## The Busy Lifestyle Factor

In today's fast-paced world, many of us are living busy lives, with little time to spare. With so much to do and so little time, it's no wonder that people often turn to convenience foods and snacks that lack nutrients. These foods are quick and easy to prepare, but they're often loaded with unhealthy fats, added sugars, and other harmful ingredients. Unfortunately, these types of food are a staple of the American diet, and they contribute to a host of health problems.

One of the main reasons why convenience foods are so prevalent in today's society is because of the fast-paced lifestyle that many people lead. With so many demands on our time, it's often difficult to find the time to cook healthy meals or to engage in physical activity. This can lead to a reliance on processed foods and snacks that are easy to grab on the go. The problem with this approach is that these foods are often high in calories, sugar, and unhealthy fats, and they provide little in the way of essential nutrients.

Another factor that contributes to the prevalence of convenience foods is the modern trend of eating out. Many people eat at restaurants or fast-food chains on a regular basis, and these establishments are known for serving large portions of food that are high in calories and unhealthy ingredients. While eating out can be a convenient way to get a quick meal, it's important to be aware of the nutritional content of the food that you're consuming.

In addition to eating out, many people rely on vending machines and convenience stores for snacks and drinks. These products are often high in sugar and other unhealthy ingredients, and they provide little in the way of nutrition. While it may be tempting to reach for a candy bar or bag of chips when you're feeling hungry, it's important to consider the long-term impact of these choices on your health.

Ultimately, the busy life factors of modern society contribute to the American diet, which is characterized by a high consumption of processed foods, unhealthy fats, added sugars, and animal products. These foods lack essential nutrients and fiber, and they can lead to imbalances in the body that cause inflammation and disease. However, by making small changes to your daily routine, it's possible to improve your diet and your overall health.

One of the easiest ways to improve your diet is to start by making small changes to your eating habits. For example, instead of reaching for a bag of chips when you're feeling hungry, try keeping a bowl of fruit or a bag of nuts on hand. These foods provide essential nutrients and are much healthier than processed snacks. You can also try packing a healthy lunch instead of eating out or reaching for convenience foods. By doing so, you can control the nutritional content of your meals and ensure that you're getting the nutrients that your body needs.

In addition to making changes to your eating habits, it's also important to find time for physical activity. Even if you have a busy schedule, it's possible to fit in a few minutes of exercise each day. For example, you can take a short walk during your lunch break or do a few minutes of stretching before you go to bed. These small changes can add up over time and have a significant impact on your overall health.

# The Solution: Moving Toward a Plant-Based Diet

In recent years, there has been a growing interest in plant-based eating as people become more aware of the impact of diet on their health and the environment. Many individuals are exploring plant-based eating patterns to improve their health, reduce their risk of chronic diseases, and lower their carbon footprint.

A plant-based diet prioritizes consuming a wide variety of whole plant-based foods, such as fruits, vegetables, grains, legumes, nuts, and seeds. This approach to eating is not only delicious but also nutrient-dense and fiber-rich. A well-planned plant-based diet can provide all the essential nutrients our bodies need and may even reduce the risk of developing chronic diseases such as heart disease, diabetes, and certain cancers.

Among their seemingly endless list of benefits, some of the most famous benefits of plant-based diets are their importance for weight management plans, heart health, and their contribution to helping us avoid developing chronic diseases.

If you have any form of concern regarding your weight management, plant-based diets might be the solution you need as they're naturally low in calories and high in fiber. In fact, they're also packed with nutrients, vitamins, and minerals, which can help you stay healthy and full of energy.

Additionally, plant-based diets have proven to be just as good alternatives for weight management as they are for heart health improvement. These wonderful natural foods can help your heart by reducing blood pressure and cholesterol levels as they're also rich in antioxidants, which can help reduce inflammation and the risk of heart disease.

Likewise, plant-based diets can also help reduce the risk of chronic diseases such as type 2 diabetes, certain types of cancer, and Alzheimer's disease. This is because plant-based diets are rich in antioxidants and phytonutrients, which can help reduce inflammation and protect against disease.

As if they weren't good enough because of their benefits to our own bodies, plant-based diets have also proven to be good for the environment. That is because they have a lower carbon footprint and require less land, water, and energy to produce. By eating a plant-based diet, you're not only helping to reduce your own risk of disease, but you're also helping to reduce the impact of food production on the environment.

You would be surprised by the number of plant-based alternatives that have the same or even more powerful effects as the most popular processed foods that have taken over supermarket shelves all over the world! For example, there are many plant-based alternatives to traditional animal products such as meat, cheese, and milk. Try swapping out traditional products for plant-based alternatives such as tofu, tempeh, nut milk, and vegan cheese.

## Magic Is Real

It's often the case that people feel like these famous plant-based diets sound like magical solutions that rarely ever live up to the expectations, regardless of how high or low those expectations may be. People tend to think that as the brain is naturally wired with the need to see before believing. Although it can be untrained from this style of thinking, in the meantime you can learn from my own story to help you believe.

My journey to a diet rich in fruits and vegetables began with a series of health problems that left me feeling lost and desperate. For years, I had suffered from severe stomach issues that had only grown worse with time. I had tried countless medications, therapies, and diets, but nothing seemed to work.

It wasn't until I began to study the science of food and its effects on the body that I realized just how important my diet was to my health and healing. I spent hours poring over medical journals, nutrition studies, and books on healthy eating, determined to find a solution to my chronic stomach problems.

At first, the thought of a diet rich in fruits and vegetables was daunting. I had always been a picky eater, sticking to my tried-and-true favorites and avoiding anything that seemed unfamiliar or unappetizing. But as I delved deeper into the science of nutrition, I began to understand just how vital these foods were to my overall health.

I started small, incorporating a handful of fruits and vegetables into each meal. I tried new recipes, experimenting with different combinations of flavors and textures. I made smoothies filled with berries and leafy greens, roasted root vegetables for a hearty side dish, and even blended cauliflower into a creamy sauce to replace my usual cheese-based options.

And as I began to eat this way, something remarkable happened. I started to enjoy these foods that had once seemed foreign and unappetizing. I found myself craving the sweetness of ripe mangoes, the crunch of fresh carrots, and the savory tang of roasted brussels sprouts. I started to feel more energized, more alert, and more alive than I had in years.

It wasn't always easy, of course. There were times when I missed my old favorites, times when I craved the comfort of a greasy burger or a cheesy pizza. But every time I gave in to those cravings, my stomach paid the price.

So, I stuck to my new diet, even when it was difficult or inconvenient. I packed my own meals when I went out with friends, brought my own snacks to work, and made sure that my pantry was stocked with plenty of fresh produce.

And as I continued to eat this way, my health began to improve. My stomach problems grew less severe, and I found myself feeling more energetic and focused than ever before. I started to see food not just as a source of pleasure, but as a source of healing and nourishment for my body and mind.

One of the turning points came when I discovered the joy of gardening. I had always loved spending time outside, but I had never considered myself much of a green thumb. But as I began to explore the world of fruits and vegetables, I found myself drawn to the idea of growing my own food.

I started small, planting a few herbs and tomatoes in pots on my balcony. But as I saw the first tender shoots of green poke through the soil, I felt a sense of excitement and pride that I had never experienced before.

Over time, my garden grew, filling my backyard with a riot of colors and textures. I grew cucumbers, zucchinis, and peppers, watching as they grew plump and ripe under the warm summer sun. I harvested juicy strawberries, sweet blueberries, and tart raspberries, savoring each bite as a taste of the earth itself.

And as I ate these foods, I found myself connecting more deeply with the natural world around me. I learned to appreciate the beauty of a sun-ripened tomato, the complexity of a freshly picked herb, and the simplicity of a crisp apple.

It wasn't just the taste, either. As I ate more fruits and vegetables, I found that my body felt more vibrant and alive. I had more energy to pursue the activities I loved, and I found myself feeling more confident and self-assured in my own skin.

Of course, as I mentioned, my journey to a diet rich in fruits and vegetables was not without its challenges. There were times when I slipped back into old habits, indulging in junk food or skipping meals in favor of convenience. But each time I did, I reminded myself of the progress I had made, and I redoubled my efforts to stay on track.

Over time, my dedication to healthy eating paid off in ways I never could have imagined. My stomach problems became a thing of the past, and I found myself feeling stronger, healthier, and more resilient than ever before.

Chapter 5:

# Plant-Powered and Perfectly Fit—

# The Wonders of a Veggie-Filled

# Lifestyle

A plant-based diet is a diet that focuses on whole, minimally processed foods like fruits, vegetables, whole grains, legumes, nuts, and seeds. By emphasizing these foods, we can increase our intake of fiber, vitamins, and minerals, while reducing our intake of saturated fats and processed foods.

One of the biggest advantages of a plant-based diet is its ability to promote better health outcomes. Research has shown that diets rich in plant-based foods can reduce the risk of chronic diseases such as heart disease, diabetes, and some forms of cancer. In addition, plant-based diets can help manage weight, improve digestion, and even promote better sleep.

But the benefits of a plant-based diet go beyond just physical health. Many people who follow a plant-based diet report feeling more energized and focused throughout the day. By eliminating heavy, processed foods that can cause energy crashes, plant-based eaters can maintain a more consistent level of energy throughout the day, leading to better productivity and focus.

Incorporating a plant-based diet into your daily routine can seem overwhelming at first, but it doesn't have to be. By focusing on whole, minimally processed foods, you can easily create a variety of delicious and satisfying meals. And by gradually incorporating more plant-based foods into your diet, you can make lasting changes that will benefit your health for years to come.

# The Nutritional Advantages of Plant-Based Diets

When it comes to nutrition, plant-based diets have numerous advantages. Eating a variety of plant-based foods provides your body with a plethora of essential nutrients, including vitamins, minerals, and antioxidants. These nutrients work together to maintain your body's health and reduce the risk of chronic diseases.

One of the most significant advantages of a plant-based diet is the abundance of vitamins and minerals. Fruits and vegetables are rich in vitamin C, which helps the body form and maintain healthy skin, cartilage, bones, and teeth. Green leafy vegetables such as spinach and kale contain vitamin K, which is crucial for blood clotting and bone health. Legumes such as beans and lentils are excellent sources of folate, a B vitamin that plays a vital role in DNA synthesis and repair. Nuts and seeds are rich in minerals such as magnesium and zinc, which are necessary for proper muscle and nerve function.

Plant-based diets are also rich in antioxidants, which help to protect your body from the damaging effects of free radicals, which are known to contribute to the development of chronic diseases. Antioxidants, such as vitamin C and beta-carotene, neutralize free radicals and help prevent cell damage. Many plant-based foods, including berries, leafy greens, and cruciferous vegetables, are rich in antioxidants.

Eating a plant-based diet has been shown to reduce the risk of chronic diseases such as heart disease and type 2 diabetes. Studies have found that a diet rich in fruits, vegetables, whole grains, and legumes can help lower blood pressure and reduce the risk of heart disease. Plant-based diets can also improve insulin sensitivity, leading to better blood sugar control and a reduced risk of developing type 2 diabetes.

In addition to reducing the risk of chronic diseases, plant-based diets can also promote healthy weight. Fruits, vegetables, and whole grains are low in calories and high in fiber, which can help you feel full and satisfied while eating fewer calories.

Overall, incorporating more plant-based foods into your diet can provide a wide range of nutritional benefits that contribute to optimal health. Whether you choose to follow a completely plant-based diet or simply increase the number of fruits, vegetables, and legumes you eat, your body will benefit from the abundance of vitamins, minerals, and antioxidants found in these foods. By nourishing your body with a plant-based diet, you can reduce your risk of chronic diseases and maintain optimal health for years to come.

# The Benefits of a Whole-Food, Plant-Based Diet

If you're looking to improve your health and overall well-being through your diet, you may have heard of various terms like whole-food, plant-based, vegetarian, or vegan diets. But what do they really mean, and how can you ensure that you're getting the most benefits from your food choices?

To answer that question, you should first have some clarity about the meaning of "whole-food, plant-based" diets. Essentially, these terms refer to a way of eating that prioritizes whole, unprocessed foods that come from plants. This means eating plenty of fruits, vegetables, whole grains, legumes, and nuts and seeds. These foods are all rich in important nutrients like vitamins, minerals, and fiber, and they're also naturally low in unhealthy fats, added sugars, and sodium.

It's important to note that whole-food, plant-based diets are different from vegetarian or vegan diets that include processed foods. Many vegetarian and vegan products on the market today, such as meat substitutes, dairy alternatives, and packaged snacks, are often highly processed and can contain large amounts of added sugars, fats, and sodium. These foods may be plant-based, but they're not necessarily whole foods, and they may not provide the same health benefits as unprocessed plant-based foods.

So, what are the benefits of a whole-food, plant-based diet? For one, it's been shown to help with weight management. Because these diets are naturally low in calories and high in fiber, they can help you feel full and satisfied while consuming fewer calories overall. This can help you lose weight or maintain a healthy weight without having to restrict your food intake or count calories.

Whole-food, plant-based diets are also great for gut health. The fiber found in these foods acts as a prebiotic, which means it helps to feed the good bacteria in your gut. This can lead to better digestion, a stronger immune system, and even improved mental health.

While you're in the process of changing your diet for the better, you should always keep in mind who you should be making this change for: *yourself.*

Take the time to understand your wants and needs, which includes being aware of your own pace. Everyone completes changes in their lives at a different pace; you just have to find yours.

Once you find it, remember to be patient with yourself. Changing your diet can be challenging, and it's important to cut yourself some slack. Don't beat yourself up if you slip up or make a less-than-healthy choice. Maintaining a healthy lifestyle is a path requiring many choices, rather than the definitive outcome of a single choice.

# Incorporating Plant-Based Foods into Your Daily Routine

Are you curious about how to incorporate more plant-based foods into your daily routine? Switching to a plant-based diet can seem intimidating at first, but with some practical tips and simple steps, it can become an enjoyable and sustainable habit.

One of the first things you can do is to start exploring new recipes and plant-based meal options. Try to find plant-based versions of your favorite meals and experiment with new flavors and textures. You might be surprised at how delicious and satisfying plant-based meals can be.

Another tip is to gradually reduce your meat and dairy consumption. You don't have to go cold turkey and completely eliminate animal products from your diet right away. Start by cutting back on the amount of meat and dairy you consume and replacing them with plant-based options. Over time, you can continue to reduce your consumption of animal products until you've transitioned to a fully plant-based diet.

It's also important to make sure that you're getting a balanced and nutritious diet. When you switch to a plant-based diet, you need to pay attention to whether you're getting enough protein, healthy fats, and essential vitamins and minerals. Incorporate a variety of whole foods into your diet, including fruits, vegetables, legumes, nuts, and whole grains. You might want to consider using a plant-based protein powder or taking a vitamin supplement to ensure that you're meeting your nutritional needs.

Another key to success is to plan and prepare your meals in advance. Set aside at least a little bit of time each week to plan out your meals and snacks and prepare them ahead of time. This can help you save time and money and ensure that you always have healthy and nutritious options on hand.

When you're eating out, don't be afraid to ask for plant-based options or make substitutions to make your meal more plant-based. Many restaurants now offer plant-based options, and you can often make simple substitutions like swapping out meat for tofu or adding extra vegetables.

As you work on changing your life for the better, remember that it's okay to make mistakes and slip up from time to time. Incorporating more plant-based foods into your diet is a journey, and it's important to be patient with and kind to yourself along the way. Have a non-plant-based meal or snack. Just acknowledge it and move on, focusing on making healthier choices in the future.

## Takeaways

It's clear that plant-based diets have many benefits for our health, the environment, and animal welfare. By incorporating more whole, plant-based foods into our daily routine, we can reap the benefits of improved digestion, better weight management, and reduced risk of chronic diseases. Plus, with the abundance of fruits, vegetables, grains, and legumes out there, there are endless delicious and nutritious options to choose from.

The transition to a plant-based diet can seem overwhelming at first, but there are plenty of practical steps you can take to make the transition easier. Start by incorporating more plant-based meals into your diet gradually, experimenting with new recipes and flavors, and focusing on whole and unprocessed foods. Don't be afraid to get creative and have fun with your food!

And remember, as with any major lifestyle change, it's important to consult with a healthcare professional to make sure you're getting all the essential nutrients your body needs. With a little planning and preparation, you can create a healthy, balanced, and delicious plant-based diet that works for you.

So, let's embrace the power of plants and take steps towards a healthier and more sustainable future. By doing so you will not simply be investing wisely in your own future, but in the future of the world as a whole!

# Chapter 6

# Nature's Healing Foods—The Power of Plant-Based Food Groups

Chronic diseases such as heart disease, diabetes, and some forms of cancer are now some of the leading causes of death in the United States. Many experts believe that our dietary choices are a major contributing factor to this trend. The standard American diet, or SAD for short, is high in processed foods, red meat, and unhealthy fats. These foods are often low in essential vitamins and minerals and have been linked to a variety of chronic health problems.

But it's not all doom and gloom. One of the most effective ways to combat chronic disease is through our diet, and a plant-based diet can play a significant role in improving our overall health. A plant-based diet emphasizes whole, unprocessed foods such as fruits, vegetables, legumes, and whole grains, while reducing or eliminating animal products and processed foods. By incorporating more plant-based foods into our diets, we can increase our intake of essential nutrients and reduce our risk of chronic diseases.

Research has shown that a plant-based diet can have significant health benefits. Studies have found that people who follow a plant-based diet have a lower risk of developing chronic diseases such as heart disease and diabetes. Plant-based diets have also been shown to help manage weight and reduce the risk of certain types of cancer.

# Leafy Greens: The Powerhouses of Plant-Based Nutrition

Leafy greens are vegetables that are, well, leafy! They're an incredibly powerful and nutritious food group that can help improve our overall health and well-being. They're generally low in calories and high in fiber, vitamins, and minerals. Leafy greens include a wide variety of greens such as spinach, kale, collard greens, arugula, and Swiss chard, to name just a few.

Eating leafy greens regularly can help prevent heart disease, type 2 diabetes, and other chronic conditions. Studies have shown that a diet rich in leafy greens can lower blood pressure, reduce inflammation, and improve glucose control, all of which contribute to a healthier heart and a lower risk of developing diabetes.

There are more leafy vegetables in this world than most of us get to see during a lifetime. However, most of us get to see some of the most useful ones a good number of times as we grow up.

For example, spinach is a great source of iron, calcium, vitamin C, and vitamin K. It's also a good source of fiber, which can help regulate digestion and prevent constipation.

Another very common one is kale. This is an excellent source of vitamin A, vitamin C, and vitamin K. It's also a good source of calcium and iron, as well as antioxidants that help fight against inflammation and disease.

Collard greens are also very famous since they're high in fiber and vitamin C, as well as calcium and vitamin K. They also contain sulforaphane, a compound that has been linked to reducing the risk of certain types of cancer.

Arugula is another must-have in your diet since it's a great source of vitamin K and folate. It also contains high levels of nitrates, which can improve blood flow and lower blood pressure.

Unsure about how to experiment with recipes that can help you make the most out of these nutritious foods? The good news is that you can literally add them to almost any type of dish. For example, you can easily add a handful of spinach or kale to your morning smoothie for a nutrient-packed breakfast.

Smoothies may seem a little too creative for some. That is why most people decide intuitively to first go for options like starting their salads with a bed of leafy greens, and then adding in other colorful vegetables and a healthy source of protein.

You can also use your leafy greens as replacements for bread and tortillas. Instead of using a wrap or bread, use a large leaf of lettuce or collard greens to make a sandwich or wrap.

Finally, you can also try sautéing leafy greens in garlic and olive oil. This is a simple and delicious way to enjoy them. You can also add other flavorful ingredients like lemon juice, red pepper flakes, or parmesan cheese.

## Berries: The Antioxidant Rich Fruit

Berries are some of the most nutrient-dense foods that nature has to offer. These delicious fruits are packed with antioxidants, fiber, and other nutrients that can offer a range of health benefits. From preventing heart disease and certain types of cancers to improving brain function, incorporating berries into your diet is an excellent way to promote overall health and wellness.

One of the most significant benefits of berries is their high antioxidant content. Antioxidants are compounds that can help protect the body against free radical damage, which can contribute to chronic diseases such as heart disease and cancer. Berries contain a wide variety of antioxidants, including vitamin C, anthocyanins, and polyphenols, all of which can help reduce inflammation and oxidative stress.

We often hear about the importance of antioxidants in our diet, but what are they exactly and why are they important? Antioxidants are compounds found in many foods that can help prevent cellular damage caused by oxidative processes. Oxidative damage is associated with aging and the development of various diseases, including cancer, heart disease, and Alzheimer's disease.

Antioxidants can protect our cells from aging by counteracting the effects of unstable molecules known as free radicals. Said molecules are neutralized when antioxidants give up electrons, keeping them from causing any damage.

Oxidative cellular processes refer to the chemical reactions that take place in cells that involve the transfer of electrons. These processes are essential for generating energy, but they also produce free radicals that can damage cells. When cells are exposed to high levels of free radicals, they can experience oxidative stress, which can lead to cellular damage and even cell death. Antioxidants help to protect cells from this damage by neutralizing free radicals.

As we age, our cells are exposed to more oxidative stress, which can lead to cellular damage and the aging process. This is because the body's ability to produce antioxidants declines with age, making cells more vulnerable to free radicals. Over time, this damage can lead to the development of chronic diseases, such as heart disease and cancer.

There are many different types of antioxidants, each with their own unique properties and benefits. Some of the most common types of antioxidants include:

- Vitamin C: This water-soluble vitamin is an important antioxidant that can be found in many fruits and vegetables, including citrus fruits, kiwi, and bell peppers. Vitamin C helps to protect cells from free radicals and can also help to regenerate other antioxidants in the body.

- Vitamin E: This fat-soluble vitamin is found in many foods, including nuts, seeds, and leafy greens. Vitamin E helps to protect cells from oxidative damage by neutralizing free radicals.

- Beta-carotene: This is a type of carotenoid, which is a pigment found in many fruits and vegetables, including carrots, sweet potatoes, and spinach. Beta-carotene can help to protect cells from free radical damage and may also have anti-inflammatory properties.

- Selenium: This is a mineral that is found in many foods, including Brazil nuts, tuna, and beef. Selenium is an important antioxidant that can help to protect cells from free radical damage and may also have anti-cancer properties.

- Polyphenols: These are a group of plant-based compounds that are found in many foods, including tea, coffee, and berries. Polyphenols can help to protect cells from oxidative damage and may also have anti-inflammatory and anti-cancer properties.

- Glutathione: This is a powerful antioxidant that is found in many cells in the body. Glutathione can help to protect cells from free radical damage and may also have anti-aging properties.

- Coenzyme Q10: This is a nutrient that is found in many foods, including fish, organ meats, and whole grains. Coenzyme Q10 is an important antioxidant that can help to protect cells from oxidative stress and may also have anti-inflammatory and anti-cancer properties.

Among the many factors that promote the oxidation of our cells, some of the most abundant and dangerous ones are known as free radicals.

Free radicals are highly reactive molecules that can damage cells, tissues, and organs by stealing electrons from other molecules in the body. They're generated during normal metabolic processes but can also be produced by external factors such as pollution, radiation, and cigarette smoke.

Free radicals affect our body through a process called oxidation that can cause damage to cells, tissues, and organs. Since these molecules lack an electron in their outer layer, they draw electrons from surrounding atoms, destabilizing them in the process.

While free radicals are a normal byproduct of cellular metabolism, they can be produced in higher quantities by external factors such as pollution, radiation, and cigarette smoke. When free radicals overwhelm the body's natural defenses, they can contribute to chronic diseases, such as cancer, heart disease, and diabetes.

It's especially important to know which types of free radicals are more concerning than others. Since they're a normal product of our metabolism and are highly present in the environment that surrounds us, the more we know about their different species, the better prepared we can be. The most concerning free radicals include the following:

- Reactive Oxygen Species (ROS): ROS are a group of free radicals derived from oxygen. They're produced as a byproduct of normal metabolic processes and can also be generated by exposure to environmental pollutants, radiation, and cigarette smoke. ROS can damage cellular structures such as proteins, lipids, and DNA, and contribute to the aging process and the development of chronic diseases.

  Antioxidants that can neutralize ROS include vitamin C, vitamin E, glutathione, and beta-carotene.

- Reactive Nitrogen Species (RNS): RNS are a group of free radicals derived from nitrogen. They're generated by the immune system to fight off invading pathogens but can also contribute to inflammation and tissue damage. RNS can damage DNA, proteins, and lipids, and are implicated in the development of chronic diseases such as cancer, diabetes, and Alzheimer's disease.

  Antioxidants that can neutralize RNS include glutathione, vitamin C, and vitamin E.

- Reactive Sulfur Species (RSS): RSS are a group of free radicals derived from sulfur. They're generated during normal metabolic processes and can also be produced by exposure to environmental pollutants, radiation, and cigarette smoke. RSS can damage cellular structures such as proteins, lipids, and DNA, and contribute to the development of chronic diseases such as cancer, heart disease, and diabetes.

Antioxidants that can neutralize RSS include alpha-lipoic acid, glutathione, and coenzyme Q10.

- Lastly, since reactive carbon species are a group of free radicals derived from carbon, antioxidants can also neutralize RCS through vitamins such as vitamins C and E, and carotenoids like beta-carotene and lycopene.

Among the many types of berries that nature can offer, you'll notice that the most accessible ones are also the ones with the most antioxidative benefits.

One of the most popular types of berries, blueberries are packed with anthocyanins, which give them their characteristic blue color. These antioxidants can help reduce inflammation, improve brain function, and lower the risk of heart disease.

Strawberries are not only as common as blueberries, but they are also a great source of vitamin C, which can help boost the immune system and improve skin health. They also contain flavonoids, which can help reduce the risk of certain types of cancers.

Another great option for your health is raspberries. These juicy berries are rich in ellagic acid, which has been shown to have anti-cancer properties. They're also high in fiber, which can promote digestive health and help manage blood sugar levels.

Blackberries do not fall behind either as they're rich in vitamin C, vitamin K, and fiber. They also contain anthocyanins, which can help reduce inflammation and improve heart health.

Regardless of the type, everyone knows berries and the many types of dishes and drinks that can stem from their amazing flavors. However, if you do not consider yourself a fruit lover or are not very experienced in these types of diets, there are some tips you may want to keep in mind.

For starters, adopting the habit of adding berries to your breakfast can change your life. Top your oatmeal or yogurt with a handful of fresh or frozen berries to start your day off with a healthy boost. However, beware as once you start you may never want to abandon this practice!

Another great way of making the most of their flavor and healing properties is to use them to make smoothies. Blend together some berries, Greek yogurt, and almond milk for a delicious and nutritious smoothie.

You do not have to be too creative with them; if you feel like you're running out of interesting ideas and want to embrace the full benefits of these foods, try snacking on them. Keep a bowl of fresh berries on hand for a healthy and convenient snack.

You have probably seen this one before but try adding them to desserts. Berries can add a natural sweetness to desserts like oatmeal bars or chia seed pudding without adding refined sugars.

## Whole Grains: The Fiber-Filled Food

Eating a diet rich in whole grains is one of the best things you can do for your health. But what exactly are whole grains? Simply put, they're grains that have not been refined and still contain all three parts of the grain: the bran, the germ, and the endosperm. Whole-grain foods are packed with nutrients that can keep your body healthy and prevent chronic diseases.

The health benefits of whole grains are numerous. One of the most significant advantages is that they can help prevent heart disease. Whole grains are rich in fiber, which can lower cholesterol levels and reduce the risk of heart disease. In addition to this, the magnesium in whole grains can also help lower blood pressure, another risk factor for heart disease.

Whole grains can also help prevent type two diabetes. Fiber slows down the absorption of carbohydrates into the bloodstream, which can prevent blood sugar spikes. Whole grains are also high in magnesium, which has been shown to improve insulin sensitivity and reduce the risk of type two diabetes.

In order to enjoy all these health benefits, you'll have to know which types of grains you should keep in your diet as much as possible. Generally, you'll notice that there are four types that can be found almost anywhere in the world and are tremendously beneficial to your health.

In the first place, you may want to try to start by including oats in your diet. They're not just one of the most accessible types of food in the world, but also are an excellent source of fiber, magnesium, and protein. They're also low on the glycemic index, which means they won't cause your blood sugar to spike.

Next, you should also keep in mind that brown rice is a great alternative to white rice. Not only is it rich in fiber, magnesium, antioxidants, and proteins, but also low in fat.

Quinoa is also a great contender for the top four most famous whole grains in the world. What makes this versatile grain so special is that it's high in protein and fiber. It's also rich in minerals like magnesium, potassium, and iron.

Lastly, when shopping for bread, look for products that are made with whole wheat. These products are an excellent source of fiber and can help keep you feeling full throughout the day.

Now that you know some of the best whole-grain foods to eat, how can you incorporate them into your diet?

Similar to berries, the use of whole grains is quite intuitive for a lot of people. However, experimenting with recipes can guarantee better results if you learn the basics of cooking with these types of foods. For example, when you're grocery shopping, choose whole-grain versions of products like bread, pasta, and rice. By swapping out refined grains for whole grains, you can boost your fiber and nutrient intake.

As you try different combinations, always remember to embrace the versatility of oatmeal as it's an easy and delicious way to incorporate whole grains into your diet. Top your oatmeal with fruit, nuts, and seeds for an added boost of nutrients.

Quinoa can work as a perfect substitute for rice. It's a versatile grain that can be often used in most of the same dishes to which you would add rice.

Finally, give yourself the liberty of snacking on some whole grains from time to time. When you're looking for a snack, choose whole-grain crackers instead of processed snacks like chips. Whole-grain crackers are a great source of fiber and can help keep you feeling full between meals.

## Legumes: The Protein-Packed Powerhouses

As we explore different ways to optimize our diets for optimal health, we cannot overlook the power of legumes. Despite being underestimated quite often, these nutritious plant-based foods offer a wide range of health benefits that are essential for our overall well-being.

Legumes are a family of plants that includes beans, lentils, chickpeas, and peas. They're high in fiber, protein, vitamins, and minerals that can improve our health in numerous ways. These nutritional powerhouses are versatile, affordable, and can be used in a variety of dishes.

One of the main benefits of legumes is their ability to improve heart health. Studies have shown that consuming legumes regularly can reduce the risk of heart disease. They're rich in soluble fiber, which can help lower cholesterol levels and improve blood pressure. Legumes are also low in saturated fat and high in unsaturated fats, which can help reduce the risk of heart disease.

Legumes are also known to have anti-cancer properties. They're high in antioxidants, which can help protect our cells from damage caused by free radicals. Additionally, legumes contain a compound called lectin, which can help prevent cancer cell growth.

Another benefit of legumes is their ability to regulate blood sugar levels. Legumes are low on the glycemic index, which means they do not cause a rapid rise in blood sugar levels. This is beneficial for people with diabetes or those who want to prevent the disease.

As has been the case with the other types of healthy types of foods discussed so far, you may be wondering what exactly legumes can replace when added to your diet and what they can smoothly blend in with. While there can be tons of different answers to this question, most opinions on the topic usually agree on the basic aspects of cooking with legumes.

The most basic and increasingly popular strategy is to use legumes in place of meat in a variety of dishes. For example, you can use black beans instead of ground beef in tacos or add chickpeas to your salads.

One of the most traditional and intuitive uses of legumes in the history of humanity is in soups. Legumes are a great addition to soups and stews. For example, you can add lentils to your vegetable soup or make a hearty chili with kidney beans.

While in some cases it may be possible for you to snack with lentils, you can take better advantage of their characteristics by eating them in hummus since this is a delicious dip made from chickpeas. It's a great snack option that is high in protein and fiber. You can dip carrots, cucumbers, or whole-grain crackers in hummus.

When it comes to using legumes, there are plenty of options to choose from but, again, you may want to start with the most popularly accepted ones since they have also proven to be extremely beneficial.

The aforementioned lentils are not just found in supermarkets and stores almost all over the globe, but they're also high in protein and fiber, making them a great addition to soups, salads, and stews.

Less popular options like chickpeas are also rich in protein, fiber, and a variety of vitamins and minerals. They can be used in hummus, salads, and soups.

Black beans are a great source of protein, fiber, and antioxidants. They can be used in a variety of dishes, including tacos, salads, and soups.

Finally, if you want to go for some lesser-known options that can rival the benefits of the other three types mentioned so far, you can try edamame. This is a type of soybean that is high in protein and fiber. It can be eaten as a snack or added to salads and stir-fries.

## Takeaways

As we wrap up this chapter on healthy foods, let's take a moment to reflect on the incredible benefits of including leafy greens, whole grains, and berries in our diets.

Leafy greens are truly one of nature's gifts, packed with a wide range of nutrients that can boost our health in many ways. Incorporating a variety of leafy greens, such as kale, spinach, collard greens, and Swiss chard, can improve heart health, reduce inflammation, and even help prevent type two diabetes. By simply adding a handful of leafy greens to our meals, we can easily increase the nutrient density of our diet.

Whole grains are another type of food that we should include more of in our diets. Unlike refined grains, which have been stripped of their fiber and nutrients, whole grains provide a wide range of health benefits. Incorporating whole grains such as oats, brown rice, quinoa, and whole wheat into our diets can improve gut health, reduce the risk of heart disease, and even help us maintain a healthy weight. Plus, with so many tasty recipes that include whole grains, it's easy to add them to our meals and snacks.

Berries are a true superfood, providing a rich source of antioxidants and other nutrients that can help protect our bodies from the damage caused by free radicals. Incorporating berries such as blueberries, strawberries, raspberries, and blackberries into our diets can improve brain function, reduce inflammation, and even help prevent certain types of cancers. Whether we enjoy them on their own or as an ingredient in a recipe, berries are a delicious and nutritious way to enhance our overall health.

While it can be tempting to rely on processed foods for convenience, these options often lack the nutritional value we need to thrive. By prioritizing natural, whole foods such as leafy greens, whole grains, and berries, we can improve our health in ways we may not have thought possible. With a little bit of creativity and planning, it's easy to incorporate these foods into our diets in a way that feels both delicious and sustainable.

# Chapter 7:

# The Hidden Hazards of Inactivity—Protecting Your Health Through Movement

*I attribute my longevity to a great extent to walking, not being in the back of the car strapped down.* —George Boggess

The benefits of exercise often tend to be underestimated. It's common for people to think that practicing exercise consistently is only for high-performance athletes or people who want to become sports superstars.

On top of that, almost everything in our modern world functions in a fast-paced way that leads us to prioritize other areas of our life over exercise. This situation has escalated to the point where many people believe that making exercise a consistent part of their daily lives will almost inevitably lead them to sacrifice a part of their income, their sleep, or even their social life.

The good news is that exercise does not have to represent a deviation from what you actually want to achieve in life, at least not if you do not want to. In fact, it's by giving into inactivity that you often put yourself at risk of not achieving your goals. The more inactive you become, the more unprepared you leave your body to face the different challenges that life will throw at you.

We have all heard the phrase "sitting is the new smoking" and, unfortunately, it's true! Physical inactivity has become a major public health problem in our modern society, and the consequences can be dire.

So, let's start with the basics: what is physical inactivity? Simply put, physical inactivity means not engaging in enough physical activity. This can include anything from sitting for long periods, such as working at a desk job, to not participating in any regular physical activity or exercise routine. In short, if you're not regularly moving your body, you're living a physically inactive lifestyle.

Physical inactivity is a growing problem in modern society, with more and more people adopting sedentary lifestyles. With the rise of technology, we're spending more time sitting in front of screens and less time moving our bodies.

The impact of physical inactivity on our health is significant. It increases the risk of chronic diseases such as heart disease, stroke, diabetes, and certain types of cancer. It also leads to weight gain, muscle loss, and a decline in bone density, which can increase the risk of falls and fractures, especially in older adults. Furthermore, physical inactivity is associated with poor mental health outcomes, such as depression and anxiety.

The good news is that physical inactivity is a preventable problem! By incorporating regular physical activity into our daily lives, we can significantly reduce the risk of chronic diseases and improve our overall health and well-being. The benefits of physical activity are numerous, from improving our cardiovascular health and reducing our risk of chronic diseases to boosting our mood and improving our sleep.

So, let's get moving! Together, we can create a healthier and happier future.

## Physical Effects of Inactivity

It's no secret that physical activity is important for our overall health and well-being. Unfortunately, physical inactivity has become a norm in our modern society. With sedentary jobs, long commutes, and technology at our fingertips, it's easy to become less active and more inactive.

When we're physically inactive, our bodies are not able to function optimally. We're more likely to develop chronic diseases and experience a decline in our physical health. Our cardiovascular health, for example, is significantly affected by physical inactivity. The heart is a muscle and, like any muscle, it needs to be worked to stay strong. When we don't engage in physical activity, our heart muscles weaken, making it harder for our heart to pump blood throughout our body. This can lead to high blood pressure, heart disease, and even stroke.

In addition to our cardiovascular health, our musculoskeletal health is impacted by physical inactivity. When we don't use our muscles regularly, they become weaker and less flexible. This can lead to a decrease in our range of motion and an increased risk of falls and injuries.

Our mental health is also affected by physical inactivity. Research shows that physical activity releases endorphins, which are natural feel-good chemicals in the brain. When we don't engage in physical activity, we miss out on these mood-boosting benefits, which can lead to feelings of stress, anxiety, and even depression.

It's important to note that physical inactivity isn't just about not exercising. It also includes sitting for long periods of time and not engaging in any physical movement. Many of us spend our workdays sitting at a desk and our leisure time sitting on the couch watching TV or scrolling through social media. This lack of movement can have serious consequences for our health.

But the good news is that even small changes can have a big impact. Incorporating physical activity into our daily routines can help mitigate the negative effects of physical inactivity. Taking short breaks throughout the day to stand up, stretch, and walk around can help increase our physical activity levels. Making a commitment to exercise regularly, even if it's just for a few minutes a day, can also help improve our overall health and well-being.

# Mental Effects of Inactivity

In today's world, physical inactivity is all too common, and its effects on our mental health are often overlooked. While it's easy to focus on the physical benefits of exercise, the mental health benefits are just as important.

Depression and anxiety are two of the most common mental health disorders, affecting millions of people worldwide. At least partly, their prevalence across the population seems to be related to physical inactivity. To understand why, it's first necessary to take a deep look at each condition.

Depression is characterized by persistent feelings of sadness, hopelessness, and a loss of interest in activities that one typically enjoys. Depression can be triggered by various factors such as genetics, life experiences, and chemical imbalances in the brain. The condition can manifest itself in different ways and may have a negative impact on various aspects of an individual's life.

Depression is more than just a feeling of sadness, and it can persist for weeks, months, or even years. It's a prevalent condition that affects millions of people globally. According to the World Health Organization (WHO), over 280 million people around the world are living with depression, and it's the leading cause of disability worldwide (*Depression*, 2021). Depression can affect people of all ages, genders, and backgrounds, and it can have severe consequences if left untreated.

The symptoms of depression can vary from person to person, and they can manifest themselves in different ways. Some of the most common symptoms of depression include: persistent feelings of sadness or emptiness, loss of interest in activities that were once enjoyed, changes in appetite and weight, difficulty sleeping or oversleeping, fatigue or loss of energy, feelings of worthlessness or guilt, and difficulty concentrating or making decisions.

Depression can affect an individual's ability to function in their daily life, including at work, in school, and in their relationships. The condition can be acute or chronic, and it can range from mild to severe. It's essential to seek professional help if you experience any symptoms of depression in order to receive the necessary treatment.

One of the most common symptoms of depression is a persistent feeling of sadness or emptiness. Individuals with depression may feel that they're not worth anything or that they have no purpose in life. These feelings can be pervasive and can impact an individual's self-esteem and confidence. People with depression may struggle with finding joy in activities that they previously enjoyed, which can lead to social isolation and a loss of interest in hobbies and passions.

Changes in appetite and weight are also common symptoms of depression. Individuals with depression may experience a loss of appetite or a desire to overeat, leading to weight changes. Additionally, changes in sleep patterns are prevalent in individuals with depression. They may have difficulty with falling asleep, staying asleep, or oversleeping. Further, many people with depression experience fatigue and loss of energy, which can make it difficult to complete daily tasks and may impact work or school performance.

Feelings of worthlessness or guilt often occur in individuals with depression. They may feel that they're a burden to others, or they may believe that they're responsible for negative events in their lives. Individuals with depression may also have difficulty concentrating or making decisions. This can impact daily tasks such as work or school assignments and can lead to procrastination or indecisiveness.

Physical inactivity also brings with it the imminent and constant threat of developing anxiety. Anxiety is a common emotional experience that most people have felt at some point in their lives. It's a natural response to stress or danger, but it can also become overwhelming and have negative effects on an individual's life as it tends to cause feelings of worry, fear, or unease.

Despite it being a normal human emotion that everyone experiences at some point in their lives, when anxiety becomes persistent and intense, it can cause disorders that interfere with daily activities, relationships, and overall quality of life.

Anxiety disorders are a group of mental health conditions that affect millions of people worldwide and can occur in people of all ages, genders, and backgrounds. They're characterized by excessive, long-term anxiety that is out of proportion to the situation at hand.

The symptoms of anxiety can vary from person to person, but some common ones include:

- Excessive worrying: A person with anxiety disorder may worry excessively about different things, such as health, work, money, or relationships. The worrying may be persistent and difficult to control, even when the individual knows that the worry is excessive.

- Irritability: Anxiety can make a person feel on edge, leading to irritability and quick tempers. This can strain relationships with friends, family, and coworkers.

- Muscle tension: Anxiety can cause physical symptoms, such as muscle tension, headaches, and fatigue. This muscle tension can cause discomfort and make it difficult to relax.

- Restlessness: Restlessness or feeling keyed up or on edge is a common symptom of anxiety. This may lead to difficulty sleeping or concentrating.

- Panic attacks: A panic attack is a sudden surge of intense fear or discomfort that can come on unexpectedly. During a panic attack, a person may feel as if they're losing control, having a heart attack, or dying. Panic attacks can be very frightening and may lead to avoiding situations that trigger them.

- Avoidance: Anxiety can lead to avoiding situations or places that trigger it. This can make it difficult to go to work, school, or social events.

- Obsessive thoughts or behaviors: Some individuals with anxiety disorders may experience obsessive thoughts or engage in repetitive behaviors to ease anxiety. These thoughts or behaviors can become time-consuming and interfere with daily life.

In addition to the increased risk of depression and anxiety, physical inactivity can also lead to decreased cognitive function. Regular exercise has been shown to improve cognitive function, memory, and overall brain health. This is because exercise increases blood flow to the brain, delivering more oxygen and nutrients that help keep the brain healthy and functioning optimally. When we don't exercise regularly, our brains don't get the blood flow they need, leading to decreased cognitive function and memory.

Physical inactivity can also lead to decreased ability to manage stress. Exercise is a natural stress-reliever, and when we don't exercise regularly, we may have a harder time managing stress in our daily lives. Exercise can help reduce cortisol levels, which is a stress hormone that can be harmful when levels are elevated for long periods. Without exercise, cortisol levels can remain elevated, leading to increased feelings of stress and anxiety.

The impact of physical inactivity can be seen in a variety of symptoms, including decreased motivation and energy, decreased productivity, and decreased self-esteem. When we don't exercise, we may not have the energy or motivation to tackle daily tasks, leading to decreased productivity and feelings of inadequacy. This can lead to a vicious cycle, where physical inactivity leads to decreased self-esteem, which can further decrease motivation to exercise.

It's important to note that the symptoms of physical inactivity are not limited to those with sedentary lifestyles. Even those who are moderately active may experience some of these symptoms if they're not getting enough exercise. This is why it's important to make exercise a regular part of our daily routine, regardless of how active we already are.

# The Importance of Regular Exercise

Regular exercise is crucial for our physical and mental health. In our modern society, physical inactivity is becoming more and more prevalent, and with it comes the negative consequences of a sedentary lifestyle. Making exercise a routine  can have a significant impact on both our physical and mental well-being.

Exercising consistently helps improve cardiovascular health. When we exercise, our heart pumps more blood, which increases the flow of oxygen and nutrients to our muscles. Over time, this can lead to a stronger heart and improved cardiovascular health. Regular exercise can also help reduce the risk of heart disease, stroke, and high blood pressure.

Regular exercise helps improve flexibility and strength. Inactivity can lead to decreased muscle strength and flexibility, which can make daily tasks more challenging and increase the risk of falls and injuries. Consistent exercise, especially strength training and stretching, can help improve our overall physical fitness and reduce the risk of injury.

It's important to note that while exercise is essential for our health, it's necessary to start slowly. For people who have been physically inactive, it's a good idea to start with low-impact activities such as walking, cycling, or swimming. As our fitness levels improve, we can gradually increase the intensity and duration of our workouts.

Finally, regular exercise can also help reduce the negative effects of physical inactivity. Inactivity can lead to a range of health problems, such as decreased cardiovascular health, weight gain, and decreased mental health. By engaging in regular physical activity, we can reduce the risk of these health problems and improve our overall physical and mental well-being.

# Discovering the Outside Again

Naturally, we tend to enjoy things more if they occur when we least expect it, and falling in love with exercise is no exception. When we try to force exercise to happen in our lives, we usually end up seeing it as a chore and a pause or distraction from a life that would otherwise be as uninterruptedly productive as possible. In fact, since exercise makes us feel tired after we practice it, when we do it because we feel we have to and not because we acknowledge its importance, we usually gain stress—instead of peace of mind—from this tiredness.

I learned this lesson the hard way with hiking. I had tried hiking in the past, but it wasn't until I had almost forgotten how it felt and decided to reconnect with the activity that I could actually make the most out of it.

I woke up one morning feeling more tired than usual. I had an extremely busy week cooped up in the press room and I could feel the weight of the stress piling up on me. I knew I needed to take a break and do something to relax.

I had always enjoyed hiking and being in nature, but I hadn't made the time for it in a while. So, I decided that it was time to change that. I packed a backpack with some essentials and headed out to one of my favorite hiking trails. The fresh air and the beautiful scenery immediately lifted my spirits. The sound of the birds singing and the rustling of the leaves in the wind were music to my ears.

As I walked, I let my thoughts wander. I realized that I had been so caught up in my work and my daily routine that I had forgotten how to appreciate the simple things in life. I had been neglecting my hobbies and passions, and it was taking a toll on my mental health. But being out in nature reminded me of the importance of taking time for myself and doing the things that made me happy.

I decided that I needed to make a conscious effort to spend more time outdoors and reconnect with my family. I had been so focused on my job that I had been neglecting my relationships. I knew that I needed to make a change if I wanted to live a more fulfilling life.

The next weekend, I invited my family to join me for a day trip to a nearby national park. We packed a picnic and set out early in the morning. As we hiked through the park, we talked and laughed and enjoyed each other's company. It felt good to be surrounded by nature and to be spending time with the people I loved.

We stopped at a beautiful spot by the river and spread out a blanket for our picnic. We sat together, enjoying the scenery and the food, and we talked about our plans for the future. It was a simple but meaningful moment, and I felt grateful for it.

After we finished our meal, we decided to explore the park some more. We found a hidden waterfall and climbed up to get a closer look. While the sound of the waterfall was deafening, I found it had a calming effect. . It was as if all my worries and stresses were being washed away by the water. I felt more at peace than I had in a long time.

As the day drew to a close, we headed back to the car. I felt a sense of contentment that I hadn't felt in a while. I realized that spending time with my family and being outdoors were two things that brought me immense joy and helped me release the stress of my busy lifestyle.

From then on, I made a conscious effort to make time for both of these things. I would take walks in the park during my lunch break at work, and I would invite my family to join me on weekend hikes. It wasn't always easy to balance my work and personal life, but I knew that it was important to prioritize the things that made me happy.

Over time, I found that being outdoors and spending time with family had a profound impact on my overall well-being. I was less stressed, more focused, and more content with my life. I realized that I didn't need to take exotic vacations or buy expensive things to be happy. All I needed was the simple pleasures of nature and the company of my loved ones.

# Chapter 8:

# Exercise for Longevity—The Connection Between Fitness and a Longer Life

Exercise has many benefits for our bodies and minds. It can improve cardiovascular health, reduce the risk of chronic diseases such as diabetes and certain types of cancer, and help us maintain a healthy weight. Exercise also boosts our mood and reduces stress, leading to better mental health and a more positive outlook on life.

Lifestyle factors such as diet and exercise play a critical role in determining our overall health and longevity. In fact, studies have shown that our lifestyle choices can have a greater impact on our lifespan than our genetic makeup. By incorporating regular exercise into our daily routine, we can significantly improve our health outcomes and increase our chances of living a long and fulfilling life.

One of the most important factors in making exercise a habit is consistency. It's essential to make exercise a regular part of our daily routine, just like brushing our teeth or getting dressed. By setting aside time for exercise each day, we can make it a priority and ensure that it becomes a regular part of our daily routine.

The good news is that exercise doesn't have to be complicated or time-consuming. Even small amounts of physical activity, such as taking a daily walk or doing a few minutes of stretching, can have significant benefits for our health. The key is to find an exercise routine that works for our individual needs and preferences, and to make it a consistent part of our daily routine.

# The Science Behind Exercise and Longevity

Exercise is essential to living a healthy, fulfilling life. It's widely known that regular exercise can help prevent many chronic diseases and improve our overall quality of life. But did you know that exercise has also been shown to increase longevity and add years to our lives?

In recent years, scientific research has shown that exercise is one of the most powerful tools we have for increasing our lifespan. Multiple studies have demonstrated that people who engage in regular physical activity tend to live longer than those who do not. In fact, research has shown that people who exercise regularly can increase their lifespan by as much as seven years!

So, what is it about exercise that makes it such a powerful tool for increasing longevity? There are several physiological processes at work that allow exercise to increase our lifespan.

One of the most important ways in which exercise improves longevity is by reducing the risk of chronic diseases. Regular exercise has been shown to lower the risk of a wide range of chronic diseases, including heart disease, stroke, diabetes, and even some forms of cancer. By reducing the risk of these diseases, exercise can help people live longer, healthier lives.

Exercise also improves cardiovascular health, which is a key factor in longevity. Physical activity increases heart rate and strengthens the heart, allowing it to pump blood more efficiently. This can help prevent heart disease and reduce the risk of other cardiovascular problems, such as high blood pressure and stroke.

Another way in which exercise promotes longevity is by reducing inflammation in the body. Chronic inflammation is a key factor in the development of many chronic diseases, including heart disease, diabetes, and cancer. Exercise has also proven to be useful in reducing inflammation in the body, which can help prevent the development of these diseases and increase lifespan.

In addition, regular exercise has been shown to improve immune function, which is another important factor in longevity. A strong immune system is essential for fighting off infections and diseases, and regular exercise is one of the best methods of improving immune function by increasing the production of white blood cells.

Exercise can also help prevent cognitive decline, which is another key factor in longevity. Studies have shown that physical activity can help preserve cognitive function as we age, reducing the risk of conditions like dementia and Alzheimer's disease.

Cognitive decline is a condition that involves a progressive loss of cognitive abilities. It's a common concern among older adults and can lead to a significant impact on their daily lives. While it's a natural part of the aging process, certain lifestyle factors, such as physical inactivity, can accelerate the decline.

Mild cognitive decline is the early stage of cognitive decline that affects memory, attention, and problem-solving skills. People with mild cognitive decline may notice a decline in their ability to remember recent events or conversations, have difficulty following complex instructions, and may struggle to solve simple problems.

The symptoms of mild cognitive decline are often subtle and can be difficult to recognize. Many people may attribute these symptoms to stress or a lack of sleep. However, if these symptoms persist or worsen over time, it's important to seek medical attention to rule out other potential causes.

When the condition escalates, it can reach the stage of severe cognitive decline, which is a more advanced stage of cognitive decline that can significantly impact a person's ability to function independently. People with severe cognitive decline may experience memory loss, confusion, difficulty with language, and have trouble with basic tasks such as getting dressed or eating.

The symptoms of severe cognitive decline are often more noticeable and can be distressing for both the person affected and their loved ones. People with severe cognitive decline may require more intensive care and support to maintain their quality of life. The following are common symptoms of cognitive decline.

- One of the most common symptoms of cognitive decline is memory loss. People with cognitive decline may forget things more frequently, especially recent events or conversations.

- Cognitive decline can affect a person's ability to communicate effectively. They may struggle to find the right words or to understand what others are saying.

- People with cognitive decline may have difficulty concentrating or may get easily distracted.

- Cognitive decline can affect a person's ability to make decisions and judgments. They may struggle to weigh the pros and cons of a situation and make an informed decision.

- Cognitive decline can make it challenging for a person to solve problems, even simple ones.

- People with cognitive decline may experience changes in their mood, such as increased anxiety, depression, or irritability.

- Cognitive decline can affect a person's ability to coordinate their movements, making it difficult to perform everyday tasks such as walking, dressing, or eating.

In addition to preventing cognitive decline, working out on a regular basis can improve overall quality of life, which is an important factor in longevity. Exercise can help people feel better, both physically and mentally, and can improve mood, reduce stress, and increase energy levels.

The good news is that it's never too late to start exercising and reap the benefits of a longer, healthier life. Even small changes in physical activity can have a big impact on longevity. Here are some tips for getting started:

- Find an activity you enjoy: The key to sticking with exercise is finding an activity that you enjoy. Whether it's walking, swimming, dancing, or gardening, find something that you look forward to doing and make it a regular part of your routine.

- Start slowly by setting realistic goals: If you're new to exercise, start slowly and gradually increase the intensity and duration of your activity. Not only will this help you to prevent injuries, but it will also allow you to stay motivated and track your progress more easily. As a result, you'll get used to practicing this habit every day of your life before you even realize it.

- Make it a habit: Make exercise a regular part of your routine. Schedule time for physical activity just like you would any other appointment or commitment.

## The Benefits of Regular Exercise

Regular exercise is one of the most important things we can do to improve our physical and mental health, and even increase our longevity. The benefits of exercise are numerous, and we can all benefit from incorporating regular physical activity into our daily routines.

If you still need some extra motivation to integrate the benefits of regular exercise into your life, you can always remember some of the most important ones discussed thus far, such as:

- Improved heart health: Cardiovascular exercise, such as running, cycling, or swimming, is great for the heart. It can help lower blood pressure, reduce the risk of heart disease, and improve overall cardiovascular health.

- Increased muscle strength and endurance: Strength training, such as lifting weights or doing bodyweight exercises, can help build muscle and increase overall strength and endurance. This can help us perform daily activities with ease and reduce the risk of injury.

- Better weight management: Exercise can help us maintain a healthy weight by burning calories and increasing metabolism. It can also help us build muscle, which burns more calories than fat.

- Reduced risk of chronic diseases: Regular exercise has been shown to reduce the risk of chronic diseases such as type 2 diabetes, certain types of cancers, and even dementia.

- Improved mood and mental health: Exercise can help boost our mood, reduce symptoms of depression and anxiety, and even improve cognitive function and memory.

- Better sleep: Regular exercise can help us fall asleep faster and improve the quality of our sleep, which can have a positive impact on our overall health.

- Increased longevity: Regular exercise has been linked to an increased lifespan. In fact, studies have shown that even small amounts of exercise can have a significant impact on longevity.

It's important to note that the type of exercise we do can impact the specific benefits we receive. Strength training, for example, can help improve muscle strength and endurance, while cardiovascular exercise can improve heart health and endurance.

In addition to the physical benefits, regular exercise can also have a positive impact on mental health by helping you prevent or reduce some symptoms of depression and anxiety. It can also improve cognitive function and memory, which can be especially important as we age.

One way exercise can impact longevity is by improving the health of our cells. Exercise can help reduce inflammation, which can contribute to a variety of chronic diseases. Exercise has also been shown to increase the production of telomeres, which are the protective caps on the ends of our chromosomes. Telomeres naturally shorten as we age, but regular exercise can help slow this process and potentially increase lifespan.

Incorporating regular exercise into our daily routines doesn't have to be complicated. Even small amounts of physical activity can have a positive impact on our health. Some ways to incorporate exercise into our daily routines include taking a brisk walk, using the stairs instead of the elevator, or doing a few bodyweight exercises during a commercial break.

It's also important to find types of exercise that we enjoy. This can help us stick to a regular exercise routine and make it a sustainable part of our daily lives. Some people may enjoy the camaraderie of a group fitness class, while others may prefer the solitude of a long run or bike ride.

In addition to the physical and mental benefits of regular exercise, it can also have a positive impact on our longevity. Even the smallest amounts of exercise can help increase your lifespan and reduce the risk of chronic diseases. By incorporating regular physical activity into our daily routines, we can improve our health and quality of life. So, let's take that first step towards a more active lifestyle and reap the benefits of regular exercise.

# Exercise and Lifestyle Factors

Living a healthy and balanced lifestyle involves taking care of different aspects of our lives, including our exercise routine and the choices we make every day. While we may not always be aware of it, our lifestyle factors have a profound effect on our overall well-being.

Lifestyle factors are the different aspects of our daily lives that can affect our physical and mental health. These can include factors such as stress, diet, sleep, and social support. When we adopt a healthy lifestyle, we make choices that can positively impact these factors, improving our overall well-being. Exercise is one such lifestyle factor that has a profound impact on our physical and mental health.

Regular exercise can help improve our stress levels, leading to a more balanced and relaxed life. Exercise accomplishes this by leading our bodies to release natural chemicals that can help alleviate stress and anxiety known as endorphins. Additionally, regular exercise can also help improve our sleep quality, leading to a more restful and refreshing night's sleep.

Diet is another important lifestyle factor that can be positively impacted by regular exercise. When we exercise, we increase our body's metabolism, which can help us burn calories more efficiently. This increased metabolism can also help regulate our appetite, leading to healthier food choices and improved nutritional intake. By incorporating regular exercise into our daily routine, we're more likely to choose healthy and nutritious food options.

Social support is another important lifestyle factor that can be improved through regular exercise. Exercise provides us with an opportunity to engage in social activities and connect with others who share similar interests. This social support can be instrumental in helping us stay motivated and committed to our exercise routine, leading to better overall health outcomes.

When we fail to prioritize exercise and other healthy lifestyle factors, we can fall into the trap of leading a sedentary lifestyle. This type of lifestyle can have a negative impact on our lifespan, increasing the risk of chronic diseases such as heart disease and diabetes. It can also lead to physical and mental health problems, including obesity, depression, and anxiety.

The good news is that we can take steps to reverse the negative effects of a sedentary lifestyle. Incorporating regular exercise into our daily routine can help improve our overall health and well-being, leading to a longer and more fulfilling life.

As you saw earlier, exercise can help alleviate stress and anxiety. This is because it triggers the release of endorphins, which are natural chemicals that can help us feel more relaxed and calm. When we exercise regularly, we may also be more likely to adopt other stress-reducing activities such as meditation and mindfulness.

Regular exercise can also help regulate our appetite and improve our metabolism. This can lead to healthier food choices and improved nutritional intake. Moreover, exercise can help boost our energy levels, leading us to feel more motivated to cook healthy meals at home instead of relying on fast food or pre-packaged options.

Exercise has also been shown to improve the quality of our sleep, and this goes beyond making us feel more tired and thus facilitating the process of falling asleep. When we exercise regularly, we're more likely to fall asleep faster and stay asleep longer. This can lead to a more restful and rejuvenating night's sleep, helping us feel more alert and energized throughout the day.

Additionally, exercise provides us with an opportunity to engage in social activities and connect with others who share similar interests. Whether we join a fitness class or participate in a running club, regular exercise can help us build a network of like-minded individuals who can provide us with support and encouragement along the way.

A sedentary lifestyle can be incredibly harmful to our health, and it's something that many of us are guilty of in our modern world. When we sit for long periods of time and fail to engage in regular physical activity, our bodies start to suffer in a number of ways. In fact, research has shown that a sedentary lifestyle can contribute to a decreased lifespan and a higher risk of chronic diseases.

When we don't move our bodies enough, our muscles start to weaken and waste away. Our bones also become weaker and more prone to fractures. This can lead to mobility issues and a decreased ability to perform everyday tasks. What's more, a sedentary lifestyle can contribute to weight gain, which can lead to a whole host of health problems, such as type 2 diabetes, heart disease, and stroke.

A sedentary lifestyle also has negative effects on our cardiovascular health. Sitting for long periods of time can lead to a buildup of plaque in our arteries, which can increase the risk of heart disease and stroke.

Additionally, when we sit for long periods of time, our blood flow slows down, which can increase the risk of blood clots.

Furthermore, a sedentary lifestyle can have a negative impact on our mental health. When we don't move our bodies enough, we may experience increased feelings of stress, anxiety, and depression. Regular exercise can help to combat these feelings, as it releases endorphins, which can help to improve mood and reduce stress.

# Making Exercise a Habit

Physical exercise is one of the most important habits we can develop to maintain a healthy lifestyle. It not only improves our physical health but also has many positive effects on our mental and emotional well-being. However, making exercise a habit is often easier said than done. It can be difficult to find the motivation to start and even harder to maintain a consistent routine.

Are you struggling to make exercise a part of your daily routine? Do you find it difficult to stick to a workout plan even though you know it's good for you? Regardless of your answers to these questions, the process of forming a new habit can be challenging for everyone. However, understanding the psychological processes that underlie habit formation can help you make exercise a natural part of your life.

To understand how habits are formed, we need to first look at the reward system in the brain. This system is responsible for the release of the neurotransmitter dopamine, which is associated with feelings of pleasure and reward. The brain releases dopamine in response to experiences that are perceived as pleasurable, such as eating delicious food, socializing with friends, or engaging in physical activity.

When it comes to exercise, the release of dopamine is particularly important because it can help create a positive association between exercise and pleasure. Over time, this positive association can help turn exercise into a habit. In fact, research has shown that individuals who exercise regularly have higher levels of dopamine receptors in the brain, which means they're more sensitive to the rewarding effects of exercise.

Another important aspect of habit formation is reinforcement. Reinforcement is a behavioral science principle that refers to the process of increasing the likelihood of a behavior by providing a reward or consequence. For example, if you want to make exercise a habit, you might give yourself a small reward every time you complete a workout. This could be something as simple as treating yourself to a healthy snack or taking a relaxing bath. Over time, this reward can help reinforce the behavior of exercise and make it more likely that you'll continue to engage in it.

It's important to note that reinforcement doesn't have to be positive. In fact, negative reinforcement can be just as effective in shaping behavior. For example, if you hate the feeling of guilt or disappointment when you skip a workout, you might use those negative emotions as a way to reinforce the behavior of exercise. This type of reinforcement is called negative reinforcement because it involves the removal of an unpleasant consequence.

So, how do habits actually form? The process of habit formation can be broken down into three main stages: a stimulus, a routine, and a reward. Any stimulus can serve as a cue that can let our brains know it's time to put a habit into practice. In the case of exercise, the cue might be putting on your workout clothes, setting your gym bag by the door, or setting a reminder on your phone to exercise at a specific time.

The routine is the behavior itself, such as going for a run or lifting weights at the gym. The reward is the positive feeling you get after completing the routine, such as a sense of accomplishment, the release of endorphins, or the satisfaction of having accomplished something that's good for your body and mind.

Over time, the repetition of the cue, routine, and reward can help cement the behavior as a habit. This is because the brain starts to associate the cue with the reward, which makes the routine feel more automatic and less effortful. This is why it's important to choose cues and rewards that are enjoyable and gratifying, as this can help make the routine feel more natural and less like a chore.

It's essential to set achievable goals when starting an exercise routine; by doing this you'll also be able to build the confidence and motivation needed to keep going until you reach your goals and beyond.

Schedule exercise time into your daily routine, just like any other appointment. Make it a non-negotiable part of your day. This will help establish exercise as a regular habit.

Partnering with someone who shares your fitness goals can be an excellent motivator. You can hold each other accountable and cheer each other on. Working out with a friend or family member can make the experience more enjoyable and increase your chances of success.

There are many fitness apps available that can help you track your progress, set goals, and create workout plans. These apps can help you stay accountable, motivated and make exercising more enjoyable.

You can literally practice exercise anywhere in the world. For many types of activities, all you need is your body! Try to find ways to be more active throughout the day. For example, take the stairs instead of the elevator, walk or bike to work, or go for a brisk walk during your lunch break. Every little bit of movement counts.

Celebrate your progress and reward yourself for meeting your exercise goals. Treat yourself to something you enjoy, such as a massage or a movie, after completing a week of consistent exercise. Making exercise a habit can be challenging, and setbacks are normal. Don't give up, even if you miss a few days or even a week. Remember that every day is a new opportunity to start fresh and keep going.

Consistency is the key to promoting longevity through exercise. The more you exercise, the more benefits you'll see, including increased muscle strength, cardiovascular health, and mental well-being. Exercise can also help reduce the risk of chronic diseases, such as heart disease, diabetes, and some types of cancer. By making exercise a regular part of your routine, you can improve your quality of life and increase your lifespan.

# Takeaways

By now, you should have a good understanding of how regular exercise can positively impact your physical and mental health, as well as your overall quality of life.

Incorporating regular exercise into your daily routine is crucial for maintaining a healthy lifestyle and improving longevity. From increasing muscle strength and flexibility to reducing the risk of chronic diseases, the benefits of exercise are clear.

It's important to remember that making exercise a habit takes time and effort. But with patience, determination, and consistency, you can establish a routine that will become a natural part of your day-to-day life.

By incorporating the tips and strategies outlined in this chapter, such as finding an exercise buddy, setting goals, and trying different types of exercise, you can find the perfect routine that fits your lifestyle and preferences.

Remember, the key to success is consistency. You can reach the point where exercise becomes a necessary part of every week, but it's wise to start by going one step at a time. Even small amounts of exercise can have a significant impact on your health and well-being, so don't be discouraged if you can't commit to long workout sessions every day.

Incorporating regular exercise into your life is a powerful investment in your future. You can reduce your risk of chronic diseases, increase your lifespan, and enjoy a higher quality of life overall. So why not start today?

Make a commitment to yourself to prioritize your health and well-being by incorporating regular exercise into your daily routine. You won't regret it.

# Chapter 9:

# Exercise for Every Body—

# Exploring the Diversity of Physical

# Activities

Regular physical activity is critical for maintaining good health and reducing the risk of chronic diseases such as heart disease, stroke, and diabetes. In this chapter, we'll explore the various types of exercise that can benefit our health, from aerobic exercise to strength training, flexibility exercise, balance training, and high-intensity interval training.

Aerobic exercise, such as running, cycling, or swimming, is excellent for improving cardiovascular health and endurance. It helps to strengthen the heart and lungs, improve circulation, and boost overall fitness levels. Aerobic exercise is also known to reduce the risk of chronic diseases such as heart disease, stroke, and diabetes.

Strength training is essential for building muscle and improving bone density. As we age, our muscles and bones can weaken, increasing the risk of falls and fractures. Strength training helps to counteract these effects by building muscle mass and bone density, improving balance and stability, and reducing the risk of injury.

Flexibility exercise, such as yoga or stretching, helps to improve joint range of motion and prevent muscle stiffness and soreness. It's an essential component of overall fitness and can help to reduce the risk of injury during other types of exercise.

Balance training is critical for improving stability and reducing the risk of falls, particularly in older adults. Exercises that challenge balance, such as standing on one leg or using a stability ball, can help to improve balance and reduce the risk of injury.

Finally, high-intensity interval training (HIIT) is a type of exercise that involves short bursts of intense activity followed by periods of rest. It's a highly effective way to improve cardiovascular fitness and burn calories, making it an excellent option for those with limited time for exercise.

## Aerobic Exercise

As humans, we were born to move. Physical activity is a fundamental aspect of our nature and essential to our overall health and well-being. Among the different types of exercise, aerobic exercise is one of the most popular and effective ways to improve our cardiovascular health, boost our endurance, and enhance our mental function.

Aerobic exercise, also known as cardio or cardiovascular exercise, refers to any physical activity that increases your heart rate and breathing rate for an extended period. In other words, it's a form of exercise that involves rhythmic, continuous movements, such as jogging, cycling, or swimming. The name "aerobic" comes from the fact that this type of exercise relies on the body's ability to use oxygen efficiently to produce energy for our muscles.

Some of the most popular forms of aerobic exercise include running, cycling, swimming, hiking, dancing, rowing, and jumping rope. These activities provide a whole range of benefits to our physical and mental health, including:

- Improved cardiovascular health: Aerobic exercise strengthens your heart and lungs, which can reduce your risk of heart disease, high blood pressure, and stroke. When you engage in aerobic activity, your heart pumps more blood and oxygen to your muscles, which can improve your overall cardiovascular fitness and endurance.

- Better weight management: Aerobic exercise can help you maintain a healthy weight by burning calories and reducing body fat. Depending on the intensity of the exercise, you can burn hundreds of calories in just 30 minutes of activity.

- Reduced stress and anxiety: As I said earlier, exercise can help your body release chemicals that can boost your mood. In fact, it can also improve your sleep, causing an even more positive impact on your mental health.

- Improved cognitive function: Aerobic exercise has been linked to better cognitive function, including improved memory, attention, and processing speed. This may be due to the increased blood flow and oxygen supply to the brain during exercise.

- Increased bone density: Aerobic exercise, especially weight-bearing activities like running and jumping, can increase bone density and reduce the risk of osteoporosis.

- Lowered risk of chronic disease: Aerobic exercise can help reduce the risk of chronic diseases, such as type 2 diabetes, certain types of cancer, and Alzheimer's disease.

- Increased lifespan: Several studies have shown that regular aerobic exercise can increase lifespan and reduce the risk of premature death from all causes.

Now that we've explored the many benefits of aerobic exercise, let's take a closer look at some of the most popular forms of cardio activity.

Running is a fantastic form of aerobic exercise that requires nothing more than a good pair of running shoes. Running can be done anywhere and is an excellent way to improve your cardiovascular fitness and burn calories. It can also be an excellent stress-reliever and mood-booster.

Cycling is a low-impact aerobic exercise that can be done outdoors or indoors on a stationary bike. Cycling is an excellent way to improve your cardiovascular fitness and lower body strength while also commuting in a way that is safe for the environment and allows you to better enjoy the fresh air that comes with each new place you'll pedal across.

Swimming is a full-body workout that provides a low-impact way to improve cardiovascular fitness, muscle strength, and flexibility. Swimming can be an excellent option for people with joint pain or injuries, and it's a fun way to cool off in the summer.

Hiking is an excellent way to get some fresh air, explore nature, and improve your cardiovascular fitness. Hiking can also be a low-impact way to improve lower body strength and balance.

## Strength Training

Strength training is an essential part of any fitness routine, providing numerous benefits to our physical and mental health. As we age, our bodies naturally lose muscle mass, which can lead to a variety of health issues such as decreased mobility, balance, and strength. By incorporating strength training into our exercise routine, we can build muscle, improve bone density, and reduce the risk of injuries.

Firstly, let's define the concept of strength training. Strength training is a type of exercise that focuses on building muscle strength, endurance, and size by working against resistance. Resistance can come from weights, resistance bands, body weight, or other types of equipment. The goal of strength training is to cause muscle hypertrophy, or an increase in muscle size, which can lead to improved strength, balance, and overall physical health.

Now that we've defined what strength training is, let's explore four examples of strength training exercises.

One of the most practiced ones both at home and in training facilities is weightlifting. This is a popular form of strength training that involves lifting weights to build muscle mass and strength. In most cases, people practice this type of exercise by using weights, such as dumbbells, barbells, or even weight machines. Weightlifting can help you build muscle and improve bone density, which can reduce the risk of fractures and osteoporosis. Additionally, weightlifting can help improve posture, balance, and coordination.

Resistance bands are also quite popular since these elastic bands come in different levels of resistance. They can be used for a variety of strength training exercises, such as bicep curls, rows, and squats. Resistance bands are portable, affordable, and easy to use, making them a great option for strength training at home or on-the-go. Like weightlifting, resistance band training can help you build muscle and improve bone density.

Similarly, you also have the option of bodyweight exercises since they use your own body weight as resistance to build strength and endurance. Bodyweight exercises are a great option for those who don't have access to equipment or prefer to exercise at home since they can also be modified to suit a variety of fitness levels. Their flexibility is due to the fact that they usually consist in exercises that demand little to no additional resources such as push-ups, squats, lunges, and planks.

Whether you're a seasoned weightlifter or a beginner just starting out, strength training can help you reach your fitness goals and improve your overall health and well-being. So, let's dive in and discover the wonderful benefits of strength training, shall we?

Strength training can help you build muscle mass and strength, leading to improved physical performance and overall health. By increasing muscle mass, you can improve balance, mobility, and coordination, reducing the risk of falls and injuries. Additionally, building strength can improve your ability to perform daily tasks, such as carrying groceries or lifting heavy objects.

As we age, our bones become more vulnerable and likely to suffer fractures and breaks since they lose a lot of their density. Strength training can help improve bone density, reducing the risk of osteoporosis and other bone-related conditions. By putting stress on the bones, strength training can stimulate the growth of new bone tissue, leading to improved bone health and a reduced risk of fractures.

By improving muscle strength, balance, and mobility, strength training can help reduce the risk of injuries. Strong muscles can help stabilize joints, reducing the risk of sprains, strains, and other injuries. Additionally, by improving balance and coordination, strength training can help reduce the risk of falls and other similar types of injuries.

## Flexibility and Balance Exercise

Exercise is not only important for building muscle or losing weight, but it's also critical for enhancing flexibility and balance. When we think of exercise, we often envision strength training or cardiovascular exercise, but it's important to remember that flexibility and balance are also crucial components of a well-rounded exercise routine.

Flexibility exercises refer to any activity that helps improve a joint's range of motion or ability to move freely. They can be static or dynamic, involve stretching or movement, and can target specific areas of the body or the entire body. Balance exercises are activities that promote stability and control of the body's center of gravity. They can improve posture, reduce the risk of falls, and enhance overall physical performance.

One of the main benefits of flexibility and balance exercises is that they help prevent injuries. When our joints and muscles are tight or immobile, we're more susceptible to sprains, strains, and other types of injuries. By improving flexibility, we can reduce the risk of injury and ensure our bodies are better equipped to handle physical activities. Additionally, balance exercises can reduce the risk of falls and improve overall stability, which is especially important as we age.

When it comes to physical fitness, it's easy to focus on strength training and cardio, but flexibility is just as important. In fact, improving your flexibility can help prevent injury, improve posture, and increase range of motion. There are several types of flexibility exercises that can help you achieve these benefits.

Yoga is a practice that combines stretching, breathing, and meditation to improve flexibility and overall well-being. It can help increase range of motion, reduce muscle stiffness, relieve tension, reduce stress, reduce anxiety, and even alleviate some depression symptoms.

Static stretching involves holding a stretch for a period of time, typically around 30 seconds. This can be done before or after a workout, and it can help improve flexibility and prevent injury.

Dynamic stretching involves moving through a range of motion, such as leg swings or arm circles. It's often used as a warm-up before a workout, as it helps increase blood flow and prepare the body for physical activity.

Pilates is a low-impact exercise that involves controlled movements and is often used for rehabilitation and injury prevention since it can strengthen your body by focusing on helping you build your core strength and improve your flexibility.

Do you ever feel unsteady on your feet or find yourself losing balance? Balance is an essential aspect of physical fitness, yet it's often overlooked. Fortunately, incorporating balance training exercises into your routine can significantly improve your stability, mobility, and overall fitness. Balance training exercises can vary from simple standing on one leg to more challenging activities, such as yoga poses, stability ball exercises, and balance board training.

Tai Chi is a gentle form of exercise that combines slow, flowing movements with deep breathing and relaxation. It's been shown to improve balance, reduce falls, and enhance overall physical function.

You can also try the intuitive and well-known technique of standing on one leg. This simple exercise involves standing on one leg for a period of time, typically 30 seconds to one minute. It can be done anywhere and can help improve balance and stability.

If it's within your possibilities, you can also try exercising with a BOSU ball. If you're not familiar with this item, it's a half-ball platform that can be used for a variety of balance exercises. It's often used in gym settings and can help improve core strength, balance, and stability.

Heel-to-toe walking is also a great way of putting your balance to the test and, thus, polishing its development. This exercise involves walking in a straight line, placing one foot directly in front of the other. It can be challenging and is a great way to improve balance and coordination.

In addition to the benefits outlined above, flexibility and balance exercises can also improve posture, reduce stress, and enhance overall physical performance. By incorporating these exercises into your regular routine, you can improve your overall physical health and reduce the risk of injury.

When it comes to flexibility and balance exercises, consistency is key. It's important to make these exercises a regular part of your routine and to continue to challenge yourself as you improve. This can be done by gradually increasing the duration or intensity of the exercise or by trying new exercises that target different areas of the body.

When it comes to learning balance and flexibility exercises, it's important to remember that everyone has a different learning curve. Some people may pick it up quickly, while others may struggle to get the hang of it. It's easy to get discouraged when you see others around you seemingly mastering a pose or movement that you just can't seem to get right. But it's important to keep in mind that we're all unique, and we all learn and progress at our own pace.

It's common to compare ourselves to others, especially in the age of social media where we're bombarded with images of people who seem to have it all together. But we need to remember that these images are often curated and don't tell the whole story. We don't see the struggles, the setbacks, and the hard work that goes into achieving these seemingly effortless poses or movements.

Learning balance and flexibility exercises can be frustrating at times, but it's important to approach it with patience, kindness, and persistence. Rome wasn't built in a day, and neither is a flexible and balanced body. It takes time and effort to get there, but the journey is just as important as the destination.

One of the keys to making progress is to focus on your own journey and not compare yourself to others. Instead, celebrate your own small victories along the way. Maybe you were able to hold a pose a little longer than the day before or touch your toes for the first time in months. These small wins may seem insignificant, but they add up and can provide the motivation to keep going.

Another important aspect of learning balance and flexibility exercises is to find what works for you. There are many different types of exercises, such as yoga, Pilates, and tai chi, and within those disciplines, there are many different styles and variations. It's important to experiment and find what resonates with you and your body. Maybe you prefer a more gentle yoga practice, or perhaps you enjoy a more dynamic and challenging Pilates routine. The key is to find what feels good for you and what you enjoy doing.

It's also important to remember that progress is not always linear. There will be times when you feel like you're taking one step forward and two steps back. That's completely normal and part of the learning process. It's important to stay committed and continue to practice regularly, even when progress seems slow or non-existent. Over time, the small steps will add up and lead to big changes.

Finally, it's important to approach learning balance and flexibility exercises with a growth mindset. This means that you view challenges and setbacks as opportunities for growth and learning. Instead of giving up when things get difficult, you see it as a chance to learn something new and improve your skills. This type of mindset can help you stay motivated and focused on your goals, even when the journey gets tough.

# High-Intensity Interval Training

High-intensity interval training (HIIT) has been gaining popularity in recent years as a fast and effective way to improve fitness levels and achieve health goals. This type of exercise involves alternating short bursts of high-intensity activity with periods of lower intensity or rest.

To begin, let's define HIIT. High-intensity interval training is a type of exercise that involves short periods of intense activity, followed by periods of rest or lower intensity exercise. These intervals can vary in length, but typically last between 30 seconds and a few minutes. The total workout time can range from as little as 10 minutes to 30 minutes or more, depending on the individual's fitness level and goals.

One of the key differences between HIIT and other types of exercise, such as steady-state cardio, is the intensity of the workout. During HIIT, the intensity is much higher, with participants pushing themselves to their limits during the high-intensity intervals. This results in a greater calorie burn and an increased metabolic rate, both during and after the workout. Another benefit of HIIT is that it can be customized to fit individual fitness levels and goals. The intervals can be adjusted to be shorter or longer, and the rest periods can be increased or decreased as needed.

Now that we have a basic understanding of what HIIT is, let's explore some examples of HIIT workouts. One popular example is sprint intervals, which involves running or sprinting for a short period of time, such as 30 seconds, followed by a period of rest or lower intensity exercise, such as jogging or walking. This cycle is repeated for a set number of rounds, usually around 10 to 15. Another example of HIIT is plyometric exercises, which involve explosive movements, such as jump squats, burpees, and box jumps, followed by a period of rest or active recovery.

Bodyweight exercises, such as mountain climbers, jumping jacks, and high knees, can also be incorporated into a HIIT workout. The key is to perform each exercise at a high intensity, with short periods of rest or active recovery in between. HIIT can also be performed with equipment, such as kettlebells or resistance bands, with exercises such as swings and snatches.

So, what are the benefits of HIIT? One of the most significant benefits is improved cardiovascular health. HIIT workouts have been shown to increase cardiovascular fitness and endurance and can also help to reduce the risk of heart disease. This is due to the fact that HIIT places a greater demand on the heart and lungs than steady-state cardio, which leads to improvements in cardiovascular function.

Another benefit of HIIT is calorie burning. Due to the high-intensity nature of the workout, HIIT can burn more calories than steady-state cardio in a shorter amount of time. In fact, research has shown that HIIT can burn up to 30% more calories than other types of exercise, such as running or cycling.

HIIT is also a fantastic way to boost metabolism since, when done properly, it often causes an afterburn effect after high-intensity intervals that lead the body to continue burning calories even after the workout is over. This is known as excess post-exercise oxygen consumption (EPOC) and can last for up to 24 hours after a HIIT workout.

HIIT can also improve insulin sensitivity, which is the body's ability to use insulin to regulate blood sugar levels. This can be especially beneficial for those with type 2 diabetes, as HIIT has been shown to improve glucose control.

When you perform high-intensity exercises, such as sprints or jumping jacks, your body's demand for energy increases rapidly. Your body then responds by breaking down stored glycogen, which is converted into glucose for energy. This process increases your metabolism, leading to a higher rate of calorie burn.

However, the benefits of HIIT don't end when you finish your workout. During the afterburn period, your body is still consuming oxygen and breaking down glycogen to fuel your recovery. This metabolic process leads to an increase in energy expenditure, even while you're at rest.

Moreover, the afterburn effect can last up to 24 hours after your HIIT workout, which means that your body is burning calories even while you're sleeping or watching TV. Therefore, incorporating HIIT into your fitness routine can be an effective way to increase your metabolism and support your weight loss goals.

In addition to the afterburn effect, HIIT also helps to increase muscle mass. This is important because muscle burns more calories at rest than fat does. Therefore, the more muscle you have, the higher your metabolism will be, even when you're not exercising.

Overall, HIIT is a great way to boost your metabolism and promote weight loss. So, if you're looking to rev up your metabolism and burn calories efficiently, give HIIT a try.

## Takeaways

It's undeniable that every type of exercise offers a vast array of benefits. Aerobic exercise, strength training, and high-intensity interval training each have their unique advantages, and it's up to us to find the type of exercise that resonates with us the most.

Whether we prefer running, weightlifting, or HIIT workouts, we all stand to benefit from regular exercise. Aerobic exercise is excellent for improving cardiovascular health, reducing the risk of chronic diseases, and boosting our overall well-being. Strength training is ideal for building muscle mass, increasing bone density, and preventing injury. And high-intensity interval training is perfect for burning calories, boosting metabolism, and improving athletic performance.

While each type of exercise offers unique benefits, what's most important is finding an exercise routine that works best for us. The fact that someone you know benefited greatly from a certain combination of exercises does not guarantee that your case will be the same. While it's always wise to seek advice from people that you trust, do it while keeping in mind that the key is to find an exercise that we enjoy and can stick to.

Incorporating exercise into our daily routines can be challenging, but it's essential for our health and well-being. By making exercise a habit, we can reap the rewards of improved physical and mental health.

In exercise, as in many other things in life, if you want to achieve positive results for your health you'll need consistency, and lots of it,—more than perfection. Even if you're doing so by taking small steps at a time, the key to success is to keep moving forward.

It's easy to get caught up in the latest fitness trends or compare ourselves to others, but we must remember that we're all on our unique fitness journeys. We must focus on our progress, no matter how small, and celebrate our victories along the way.

# Conclusion

Remember, living a healthy lifestyle isn't about perfection or deprivation. It's about making small, sustainable changes that will benefit your mind, body, and soul. It's about finding the joy in movement, the nourishment in food, and the peace in mindfulness.

I encourage you to start with small changes that fit your life and your goals, whether that means adding more vegetables to your diet, taking a daily walk, or incorporating meditation into your routine. Over time, these small steps can lead to big transformations and lasting health benefits.

Above all, remember that your health is worth investing in. You're worth investing in. Your life is a precious gift, and taking care of yourself will allow you to live it to the fullest. So, go forth, be kind to yourself, and enjoy the journey towards a healthy and fulfilling life.

While we have discussed many topics related to healthy living, such as stress management, healthy diets, and physical activity, there are still many challenges to overcome.

Stress is one of the biggest threats to our health and well-being. It can affect all aspects of our lives, including our mental, emotional, and physical health. Chronic stress can lead to numerous health problems such as cardiovascular disease, immune dysfunction, and cognitive decline. But the good news is that we can take steps to manage our stress and reduce its impact on our health. Techniques such as mindfulness, meditation, yoga, and exercise can help us manage stress and live a healthier, more balanced life.

Unhealthy diets are another major threat to our health. Diets high in processed foods, sugar, and saturated fat can lead to chronic diseases such as obesity, type 2 diabetes, and heart disease. By contrast, plant-based diets that are high in whole grains, fruits, and vegetables have been shown to promote health and reduce the risk of chronic disease.

By making small changes to our diet, such as replacing processed snacks with fresh fruits or swapping meat for plant-based proteins, we can make a big difference in our health.

Physical inactivity is another major threat to our health. A sedentary lifestyle can lead to a range of health problems such as obesity, cardiovascular disease, and cognitive decline. But the good news is that we can incorporate physical activity into our daily routine in many ways, such as walking, cycling, swimming, or even dancing. By finding an activity that we enjoy and making it a regular part of our lives, we can improve our health, reduce our risk of chronic disease, and enhance our quality of life.

Living an unhealthy life can be a very self-destructive experience, both physically and emotionally. The lack of energy and motivation, the chronic illnesses and pain, the feelings of stress and anxiety, can all add up to a bleak existence.

But, conversely, living a healthy life can be a truly amazing experience. It's not just about the physical benefits, such as increased energy, improved mood, and a reduced risk of chronic diseases. It's about the sense of empowerment, the feeling of control over your life, the confidence and self-respect that comes from making choices that honor your body and mind.

Living a healthy lifestyle means choosing to be the best version of yourself, and that's an incredibly powerful feeling. It means nourishing your body with wholesome, nutritious foods, staying active, and taking care of your mental health. It means prioritizing self-care and making choices that align with your values and goals.

The truth is, no one can make these choices for us. It's up to each of us to take responsibility for our own health and well-being. It's up to us to decide that we're worth the effort, that we deserve to feel our best, and that we're capable of making positive changes in our lives.

So, as you embark on this journey towards a healthy lifestyle, remember that it's not just about the destination. It's about the journey itself, the small steps that you take each day towards a healthier, happier life. It's about finding joy in the process, and celebrating every victory, no matter how small.

And always remember, you're not alone. There are countless resources available to help you along the way, from fitness classes and support groups to online communities and wellness coaches. The most important thing is to keep moving forward, and to never give up on yourself.

In the end, living a healthy lifestyle is not just a goal, but a way of life. It's about embracing the journey, making mindful choices, and nurturing your body and mind. So, go forth and live your best life, and know that the journey is well worth it.

# References


*Aerobic exercise health information.* (2019, July 16).Cleveland Clinic. https://my.clevelandclinic.org/health/articles/7050-aerobic-exercise

*Anniversary messages.* (n.d.) The Royal Family. https://www.royal.uk/anniversary-messages-0

*Antioxidants: Beyond the hype.* (2012, September 18). Harvard School of Public Health. https://www.hsph.harvard.edu/nutritionsource/antioxidants/

*Antioxidants.* (2019). MDPI. https://www.mdpi.com/journal/antioxidants

Aubrey, A. (2022, August 31). *The U.S. diet is deadly. Here are 7 ideas to get Americans eating healthier.* NPR. https://www.npr.org/sections/health-shots/2022/08/31/1120004717/the-u-s-diet-is-deadly-here-are-7-ideas-to-get-americans-eating-healthier

Belzile, L. R. (2022, December 6). *Heads or tails: What statistical models tell us about the probability of living beyond 110.* The Conversation. https://theconversation.com/heads-or-tails-what-statistical-models-tell-us-about-the-probability-of-living-beyond-110-189287

Biddulph, M.. (2022, November 3). *Plant-based diet: What to eat, health benefits and tips.* Livescience. https://www.livescience.com/plant-based-diet

*Brain basics: Reward system drives our behaviour.* (n.d.) The Reward Foundation. https://rewardfoundation.org/brain-basics/reward-system/

Buchholz, K. (2021, February 5). *Is 100 the new 80? Centenarians are becoming more common.* Statista. statista.com/chart/18826/number-of-hundred-year-olds-centenarians-worldwide/

Cardiovascular diseases. (2021, June 11). World Health Organization. https://www.who.int/news-room/fact-sheets/detail/cardiovascular-diseases-(cvds)#:~:text=Cardiovascular%20diseases%20(CVDs)%20are%20the,%2D%20and%20middle%2Dincome%20countries.

Cherry, K. (2019, November 8). *How our brain neurons can change over time from life's experience.* Verywell Mind. https://www.verywellmind.com/what-is-brain-plasticity-2794886

Chu, B., Marwaha, K., & Ayers, D. (2022, September 12). *Physiology, stress reaction.* PubMed; StatPearls Publishing. https://www.ncbi.nlm.nih.gov/books/NBK541120/

*Depression* (2021, September 13). World Health Organization. https://www.who.int/news-room/fact-sheets/detail/depression

*Diagnostic and statistical manual of mental disorders DSM-5 TM.* (2013). American Psychiatric Association. https://cdn.website-editor.net/30f11123991548a0af708722d458e476/files/uploaded/DSM%2520V.pdf

Dolgin, E. (2018). *There's no limit to longevity, says study that revives human lifespan debate. Nature, 559*(7712), 14–15. https://doi.org/10.1038/d41586-018-05582-3

Dunsky, A. (2019). The effect of balance and coordination exercises on quality of life in older adults: A mini-review. *Frontiers in Aging Neuroscience, 11*(318). https://doi.org/10.3389/fnagi.2019.00318

Eagleson, C., Hayes, S., Mathews, A., Perman, G., & Hirsch, C. R. (2016). The power of positive thinking: Pathological worry is reduced by thought replacement in Generalized Anxiety

Disorder. *Behaviour Research and Therapy, 78*, 13–18. https://doi.org/10.1016/j.brat.2015.12.017

Emilio, E. J. M.-L., Hita-Contreras, F., Jiménez-Lara, P. M., Latorre-Román, P., & Martínez-Amat, A. (2014). The association of flexibility, balance, and lumbar strength with balance ability: Risk of falls in older adults. *Journal of Sports Science & Medicine, 13*(2), 349–357. https://www.ncbi.nlm.nih.gov/pmc/articles/PMC3990889/

Fairbank, R. (2022, August 24). People who do strength training live longer—and better. *The New York Times.* https://www.nytimes.com/2022/08/24/well/move/cardio-strength-training-benefits.html

Fletcher, J. (2022, July 8). *Balance exercises: Types, benefits, and more.* Medical News Today.https://www.medicalnewstoday.com/articles/balance-exercises

Graber, E. (2022, July 28). *ASN journals examine health benefits of plant-based diets.* American Society for Nutrition. https://nutrition.org/asn-journals-examine-health-benefits-of-plant-based-diets/

Guy-Evans, O. (2021, March 11). *Central nervous system (CNS) structure and function.* Simply Psychology. https://www.simplypsychology.org/central-nervous-system.html

Guy-Evans, O. (2021, July 8). *Brain reward system.* Simply Psychology. https://www.simplypsychology.org/brain-reward-system.html

Herman, J. P., McKlveen, J. M., Ghosal, S., Kopp, B., Wulsin, A., Makinson, R., Scheimann, J., & Myers, B. (2016). Regulation of the hypothalamic-pituitary-adrenocortical stress response. *Comprehensive Physiology, 6*(2), 603–621. https://doi.org/10.1002/cphy.c150015

Hinds, J. A., & Sanchez, E. R. (2022). The role of the hypothalamus–pituitary–adrenal (HPA) axis in test-induced anxiety: Assessments, physiological responses, and molecular details. *Stresses, 2*(1), 146–155. https://doi.org/10.3390/stresses2010011

Iliades, C. (2021, October 5). *The benefits of strength and weight training.* Everyday Health.https://www.everydayhealth.com/fitness/add-strength-training-to-your-workout.aspx

Kandola, A. (2019, November 22). *Aerobic exercise: Benefits for the body and the brain.* Medical News Today.https://www.medicalnewstoday.com/articles/327100

*Know your brain: Reward system.* (n.d.) Neurochallenged. https://neuroscientificallychallenged.com/posts/know-your-brain-reward-system

Lewis, R. G., Florio, E., Punzo, D., & Borrelli, E. (2021). The brain's reward system in health and disease. *Advances in Experimental Medicine and Biology, 1344,* 57–69. https://doi.org/10.1007/978-3-030-81147-1_4

Lobo, V., Patil, A., Phatak, A., & Chandra, N. (2010). Free radicals, antioxidants and functional foods: Impact on human health. *Pharmacognosy Reviews, 4*(8), 118–126. https://www.ncbi.nlm.nih.gov/pmc/articles/PMC3249911/

Mayo Clinic Staff. (2021, May 15). *Strength training: Get stronger, leaner, healthier.* Mayo Clinic. https://www.mayoclinic.org/healthy-lifestyle/fitness/in-depth/strength-training/art-20046670

Mayo Clinic Staff. (2022, February 3). *Positive thinking: Stop negative self-talk to reduce stress.* Mayo Clinic. https://www.mayoclinic.org/healthy-lifestyle/stress-management/in-depth/positive-thinking/art-20043950

Mersy, D. J. (1991). Health benefits of aerobic exercise. *Postgraduate Medicine, 90*(1), 103–107, 110–112. https://doi.org/10.1080/00325481.1991.11700983

Patel, H., Alkhawam, H., Madanieh, R., Shah, N., Kosmas, C. E., & Vittorio, T. J. (2017). Aerobic vs anaerobic exercise training effects on the cardiovascular system. *World Journal of Cardiology, 9*(2), 134. https://doi.org/10.4330/wjc.v9.i2.134

Puderbaugh, M., & Emmady, P. (2022, May 8). *Neuroplasticity.* StatPearls. https://www.statpearls.com/ArticleLibrary/viewarticle/97078

Rapaport, L. (2022, December 12). *Quick bursts of intense physical activity may help you live longer.* EverydayHealth. https://www.everydayhealth.com/longevity/quick-bursts-of-intense-physical-activity-may-help-you-live-longer/

Shaffer, J. (2016). Neuroplasticity and clinical practice: Building brain power for health. *Frontiers in Psychology, 7*(1118). https://doi.org/10.3389/fpsyg.2016.01118

Shokrpour, N., Sheidaie, S., Amirkhani, M., Bazrafkan, L., & Modreki, A. (2021). Effect of positive thinking training on stress, anxiety, depression, and quality of life among hemodialysis patients: A randomized controlled clinical trial. *Journal of Education and Health Promotion, 10,* 225. https://doi.org/10.4103/jehp.jehp_1120_20

Sissons, B. (2019, August 29). *Plant based diet: A guide for health and nutrition.* Medical News Today. https://www.medicalnewstoday.com/articles/326176

Smith, S. M., & Vale, W.W. (2006). The role of the hypothalamic-pituitary-adrenal axis in neuroendocrine responses to stress. *Dialogues in Clinical Neuroscience, 8*(4), 383–395. doi: https://doi.org/10.31887/DCNS.2006.8.4/ssmith

Storey, A. (2021, September 23). *Estimates of the very old, including centenarians, UK: 2002 to 2020.* UK Office of National Statistics.

https://www.ons.gov.uk/peoplepopulationandcommunity/birt
hsdeathsandmarriages/ageing/bulletins/estimatesoftheveryoldi
ncludingcentenarians/2002to2020

*Strength training builds more than muscles.*(2021, October 13). Harvard Health Publishing. https://www.health.harvard.edu/staying-healthy/strength-training-builds-more-than-muscles

*The power of positive thinking.* (2019). Johns Hopkins Medicine Health Library. https://www.hopkinsmedicine.org/health/wellness-and-prevention/the-power-of-positive-thinking

Tuso, P., Ismail, M., Ha, B., & Bartolotto, C. (2013). Nutritional update for physicians: Plant-based diets. *The Permanente Journal, 17*(2), 61–66. https://doi.org/10.7812/tpp/12-085

*Understanding the stress response.* (2020, July 6). Harvard Health Publishing. https://www.health.harvard.edu/staying-healthy/understanding-the-stress-response

Walker, C. (2015). The effects of an American diet on health. *Inquiro:Journal of UAB's Undergraduate Research Journal, 9.* https://www.uab.edu/inquiro/issues/past-issues/volume-9/the-effects-of-an-american-diet-on-health

Wartella, E. A., Lichtenstein, A. H., & Boon, C. S. (Eds). (2010). *Overview of health and diet in America.* National Academies Press. https://www.ncbi.nlm.nih.gov/books/NBK209844/

*Why balance and flexibility training are essential to balanced fitness—Part 2.* (2022, February 28). Biostrap. https://biostrap.com/academy/why-balance-and-flexibility-training-are-essential-to-balanced-fitness-part-2/

Wilson, M. M., Reedy, J., & Krebs-Smith, S. M. (2016). American diet quality: Where it is, where it is heading, and what it could be. *Journal of the Academy of Nutrition and Dietetics, 116*(2), 302-310.e1. https://doi.org/10.1016/j.jand.2015.09.020

Yaribeygi, H., Panahi, Y., Sahraei, H., Johnston, T. P., & Sahebkar, A. (2017). The impact of stress on body function: A review.

*EXCLI Journal,* *16*(1), 1057–1072. https://doi.org/10.17179/excli2017-480